Psychology of Behaviour Restrictions and Public Compliance in the Pandemic

This volume examines the topic of compliance with COVID-19 restrictions, and the non-pharmaceutical measures taken by governments in attempts to bring the pandemic under control.

Discovery that COVID-19 was largely transmitted through the air meant that public health strategies were needed to limit close physical contact between people. Epidemiological modelling offered initial interventions to tackle the rate of spread, but to be effective these measures were dependent on widespread public adoption and compliance. This book examines the key theories and empirical approaches to behavioural change and compliance, and reviews research on their relative effectiveness in driving public behaviour. Author Barrie Gunter considers four principal models used: nudge theory, social identity-group processes theory, theory of planned behaviour and the capability-opportunity-motivation-behaviour (COM-B) model. Gunter weighs the pros and cons of each, offers commentary on lessons that can be learned from their application during the pandemic, and what they may have to offer in a triangulated approach, theoretically, methodologically and in terms of policy making.

Examining not just the extent of compliance but also the psychological drivers of this behaviour over time, this is essential reading for students and researchers in psychology, public health and medical sciences, and policy makers assessing government strategies, responses and performance.

Barrie Gunter is Emeritus Professor in Media at the University of Leicester, UK. A psychologist by training, he has published more than 80 books on a range of media, marketing, business, leisure and psychology topics.

Psychology of Behaviour Restrictions and Public Compliance in the Pandemic

Lessons from COVID-19

Barrie Gunter

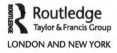
LONDON AND NEW YORK

Cover image: Getty Images

First published 2022
by Routledge
4 Park Square, Milton Park, Abingdon, Oxon OX14 4RN

and by Routledge
605 Third Avenue, New York, NY 10158

Routledge is an imprint of the Taylor & Francis Group, an informa business

British Library Cataloguing-in-Publication Data
A catalogue record for this book is available from the British Library

Library of Congress Cataloging-in-Publication Data
A catalog record has been requested for this book

ISBN: 978-1-032-22817-4 (hbk)
ISBN: 978-1-032-22815-0 (pbk)
ISBN: 978-1-003-27430-8 (ebk)

DOI: 10.4324/9781003274308

Typeset in Sabon
by MPS Limited, Dehradun

Contents

Contents

Chapter 1

Pandemic Strategy and Public Behaviour

The coronavirus pandemic was the biggest health crisis and international emergency the world had faced in peacetime for 100 years. It was certainly the biggest national catastrophe in the United Kingdom outside the Second World War. In the absence of tried and tested medical treatments or vaccines to protect their populations against this new virus, governments and their public health authorities had to turn to "non-pharmaceutical interventions" (NPIs). Essentially these methods comprised a number of behavioural restrictions and recommended personal protection measures. The behavioural restrictions, to be effective against a highly infectious new disease, had to be far-reaching and in many cases legally enforced. In effect, they resulted in the closure of many aspects of national economies and societies. Public compliance with the restrictions tended to be widespread, and most recommended actions were adopted by most of the people. In the early stages of the ensuing pandemic, people were generally understanding about why they needed to obey the requests and instructions of their government. Over time, in relation to some behaviours, public patience was tested.

There is no doubt that many governments were caught napping by the speed with which this pandemic spread around the world and especially among their populations. Many were caught ill-prepared to cope with a health crisis on this scale. Inevitably, questions were asked about government's strategies and decision making in relation to the policies they adopted and enacted to tackle the emergency they faced. Finding fault and allocating blame were two natural reactions in this context that were frequently magnified, if not created, by media commentaries and analyses.

Always needed were clearly thought-out and articulated explanations of what was known and what was unknown about this new virus and about which intervention measures appeared to work well or less well to bring the pandemic under control. Lessons needed to be learned and were learned. Yet, too often, decision-makers shot themselves in the foot or created unnecessary confusion among the public by fudging, falsifying, over-promising and getting things wrong.

DOI: 10.4324/9781003274308-1

Although the political defence, often sounded, that it was easy after the fact to criticise public policy decisions with the benefit of hindsight, it is equally reasonable and true to say that experts in a number of fields of medical science had a background of knowledge about epidemics and pandemics, their causes, their cures and ways to control them with NPIs (Bootsma & Ferguson, 2007; Mackenzie, 2020).

A global pandemic on the scale of the one caused by the SARS-CoV-2 virus may have been a "once in a lifetime" event, but it was not unprecedented (Heneghan & Jefferson, 2020; Menachery et al., 2016). Some writers gave warnings of an imminent global pandemic crisis less than two years before the 2020–2021 pandemic (FEMA, 2019; McGrath, 2019; Yong, 2018). Lessons of relevance to the pandemic of 2020–2021 were still learned and written about in the 21st century concerning the Spanish influenza pandemic of 1918–1920 (Barry, 2004; Jeffery & David, 2006). Other pan-national but globally less impactful coronavirus and influenza outbreaks had also occurred in the 21st century giving countries most affected some advance knowledge that could have served them well when confronted with COVID-19 (Henig, 2020).

An outbreak of swine flu or H1N1 in 2009–2010 surfaced in Mexico in April 2009 and spread globally leading it to be classified as a pandemic. In this case, young people were the ones most at risk, whereas older people were more likely to have some immunity to it gained from earlier influenza viruses. It was declared officially over by August 2010 and now there is a suite of flu vaccines that are widely available every year for administration prior to seasonal flu outbreaks. Swine flu was estimated to have caused, worldwide, between 150,000 and 575,000 deaths, of which eight in ten occurred among the under-65s (Heneghan & Jefferson, 2020).

There were just 138 deaths attributed to swine flu in England between June and November 2020. Around 540,000 had been estimated to have symptoms of influenza in England during this period (NHS, 2009). There had been no deaths in the United Kingdom from SARS-CoV-1 or Middle East respiratory syndrome (MERS). Hence, recent pandemics had not really affected Britain. Given the pandemic experiences of other parts of the world during the 21st century and the longer history of managing them dating back to the 19th century, there was really no excuse for the government and National Health Service not being prepared to deal with a major outbreak of a new and infectious virus (Bootsma & Ferguson, 2007; Jeffery & David, 2006; Kalnins, 2006; Markel et al., 2007).

Yet, the relatively minor impacts of recent outbreaks on the United Kingdom perhaps offer some explanation as to why the SARS-CoV-2 outbreak was not something treated with any sense of urgency by the British government. Until that is the emergence of epidemiological modelling that projected up to half a million British deaths from this new virus if it was left to spread unchecked (Flaxman et al., 2020).

For the most part, it is probably reasonable to assume that those in government and those in the most senior management positions in the myriad public health, clinical/medical and other scientific bodies engaged in fighting this new and highly infectious disease meant well and tried to do the best they could, within the constraints of their knowledge at the time and resources at their disposal, to put in place effective strategies designed to protect the public. Just how effectively governments performed is a matter that will become clearer with the passage of time and with follow-up public inquiries once the SARS-CoV-2 pandemic has been brought under control.

Many different scientific disciplines were activated during the 2020–2021 pandemic. These included various medical sciences involved in developing vaccines, therapies and treatments, and understanding at a microscopic level, the structure of the virus and how it infects people. Then there were physical sciences and engineering experts that studied how viral particles moved around in different physical settings and what kinds of mitigating physical interventions could be deployed, such as coverings and screens and ventilation and air purifying systems, to reduce viral transmissions.

Finally, there were social and behavioural sciences that played an important part in understanding which behaviour control and protective measures would be accepted or rejected by people. The latter measures played a critical role in controlling viral transmission throughout the pandemic but especially so during the early months after outbreaks had occurred given that pharmaceutical or medical sources of protection were non-existent or in short supply. This book focuses on behavioural interventions and behavioural adoption of some pharmaceutical developments, most notably vaccines.

From Epidemiology to Behavioural Modelling

At the outset of the pandemic, the absence of approved vaccines or tried-and-tested drug treatments for COVID-19 meant that governments and their public health authorities had to be reliant on other measures, collectively labelled as "non-pharmaceutical interventions" or NPIs to bring accelerating rates of virus transmission under control. These NPIs comprised the adoption of new behaviour patterns. These included the adoption of enhanced personal protective measures such as regular handwashing and the wearing of face masks. Mostly, though, the restrictions centred on keeping people physically apart. This was an obvious step to take once it had been established by medical experts that COVID-19 was mainly an airborne disease.

Initial epidemiological modelling predicted the short-term effects of specific interventions on infection transmission rates such as shop closures, school closures, workplace closures, stay-at-home warnings, reductions in traffic levels on public transport and implementation of social distancing advisories. Ultimately, they were concerned with the prediction of human behaviour patterns. Early models were able to predict viral transmission levels that would occur over a specific designated time period with and without the implementation of these interventions. One such model persuaded the British government dramatically to change its strategy for managing the early pandemic by locking down much of the UK economy and society (Flaxman et al., 2020).

These epidemiological models had a powerful influence over early government pandemic strategies. What those models did not provide much evidence about was how people would behave under these changed circumstances. To know more about behaviour control it is essential to turn to behavioural sciences, including psychology (Arnot et al., 2020).

Telling people to stay home and not to see other people is easy enough to say but presents many significant challenges in terms of behavioural compliance. Human beings are naturally social animals. They have to be to maintain the species. In evolutionary terms, humans must interact with others to find mates and to procreate the species. This act grows out of social interactions in which social relationships become established. To diversify the gene pool, it became essential for individuals to look beyond their own immediate communities and this meant going out and about to find partners with whom to procreate. This behavioural characteristic of venturing out to meet other people has therefore been conditioned in the human species over millennia.

The success of this approach to "flattening the curve" of rising infection rates was dependent upon people playing along and doing their part. Public compliance with the restrictions was crucial. In some ways, people were given no choice when governments closed down many of the spaces in which they normally interacted such as schools and universities, bars, cafes and restaurants, gyms and social clubs, entertainment and sports events, and most retail outlets. The government also asked people to work from home and for employers to encourage this behaviour wherever possible. These restrictions also mandated that people from different households should not inter-mingle. Furthermore, people should only leave home for essential reasons such as shopping for food and medicines and for taking exercise. The latter restrictions could not always be policed by the authorities and therefore depended upon people voluntarily complying (Cook, Zhao, Chen & Finkelstein, 2018).

While epidemiologists had produced modelling that advised governments to deploy these interventions to control COVID-19 transmission rates, they were not able to show through their models whether people would be compliant. A different kind of analysis was required to demonstrate the likelihood that this would happen. The discipline of psychology was centre-stage at this point. It had models that could predict or explain how public behaviour control might be achievable. None of the available or most popularly used models of this sort could be deemed to be perfect. Nevertheless, they were capable of underpinning the design of empirical inquiries that could produce data to indicate how people's normal behaviour patterns might be changed.

This book will examine public compliance with behavioural restrictions deployed by governments during the COVID-19 pandemic. Four principal psychological models will be considered. There are other theories from psychology that can be used to investigate behaviour change under circumstances like this, but the ones put under the microscope here were widely used by researchers around the world who investigated peoples' behavioural compliance during the pandemic.

The four theoretical frameworks are nudge theory, social identity/group process theory, the theory of planned behaviour and the compatibility-opportunity-motivation-behaviour (COM-B) model. Each of these approaches was used by researchers to investigate people's reactions to the pandemic and its associated behavioural restrictions. Subsequent chapters will tease out how useful these theories turned out to be in more detail by drawing upon illustrative studies from around the world.

The four models derive from two general approaches to behaviour change. These have been labelled by some as "instrumental compliance" and "normative compliance" (Neville et al., 2021). The instrumental approach is characterised by the use of direct interventions that require people to change their behaviour and use sanctions or penalties to encourage people to be compliant and to frighten them out of disobeying newly imposed rules and regulations governing public conduct. Authorities issue instructions, guidance and recommendations to the public but ensuring compliance must also create a system of monitoring how people behave in order to identify miscreants.

People might feel threatened by behaviour change interventions following this approach, but might be tempted to breach what they have been told to do if they believe they can get away with it. In other words, behavioural restrictions that are externally imposed must be externally enforced and often will not be internalised by people. Resistance to behavioural restrictions can be especially likely to occur when public do not like or trust their authorities, when important membership or reference groups encourage disobedience or non-compliance, or when compliance causes damaging side effects they cannot tolerate (Bonell et al., 2020; Haslam et al., 2018; Bavel et al., 2020). In contrast, normative compliance approach will use more subtle techniques to get people to change their behaviour by gently nudging them towards a desired behaviour or by creating conditions socially in which others who represent important sources of influence are encouraged to adopt new norms of behaviour.

Tackling the Pandemic in Britain: Early Psychology

In the United Kingdom, the principal messaging, at the outset of the pandemic, focused most on "protecting the National Health Service". This message was grounded in the need to bring under control the rapidly growing numbers of people that developed symptoms severe enough to warrant admission to hospital. There were no known vaccines or drug treatments for this new virus available when the disease first spread around the world. Health authorities worried that this disease could overwhelm hospital capacities even in those countries with the best-resourced health systems.

Further messaging about the pandemic made it clear that everyone had a part to play. This was understandable given that in the absence of medical interventions, non-medical or NPIs were needed instead. The position became clear very quickly, despite the delays in some countries in acting as robustly as they could when initially confronted with this new disease. The public could not simply sit back and wait for the authorities to sort things out. More than that, the public *should not expect* the authorities alone to save them. It was essential and therefore reasonable for the authorities to call upon everyone to become stakeholders in the process of combating this new disease.

Initially, messaging from the government in the United Kingdom was that light-touch interventions might suffice to bring the virus under control. There was much focus on personal cleanliness. People were told to wash their hands regularly. They were told to resist touching their faces. They were to avoid touching surfaces when out and about (e.g., visiting the shops, travelling on public transport) and to sanitise their hands once they had completed their journey. There was also a big push of washing down surfaces that people might touch. This approach was guided by "nudge theory". This approach, which is explained more fully later on, focused on providing the public with regular and often subtle signals in their everyday environments that were designed to direct their behaviour. Sometimes these signals appeared as physical signs such as advisory warnings, floor markings, and messages through the media that tried to influence personal risk perceptions and fears.

None of these early measures or requests was that onerous. They could easily be adopted by everyone – although with some additional cost in relation to purchasing sanitisers, soaps, cleaning materials and so on. These interventions were grounded in the belief that surface transmission of the virus was a major factor in its spread. Then, two important discoveries were made that changed pandemic control strategy. First, there was the discovery that the novel coronavirus was mostly transmitted in the air by infected people giving it to the uninfected when they shared the same breathing space and found themselves in close enough proximity for more than a critical period of time.

Second, it was also found that a significant proportion of people who caught the virus were asymptomatic and did not know they had caught it or had only mild symptoms which they dismissed as something else such as a common cold. This meant that it was not always possible to determine, from external appearances only, who had caught the disease and who had not. Only clinical testing could resolve this problem and at the outset effective and accurate tests for COVID-19 infection were not available or certainly not at mass testing scale.

All this meant that NPIs were crucial. Furthermore, to be really effective on a population-wide basis, given the infectiousness of the new virus and the complications caused by it being airborne, only comprehensive shutting down of most human-to-human physical and social contact was likely to be effective in "flattening the curve" or rapidly rising infections and hospitalisations. Some governments recognised this position quicker than others. A few such as Italy and Spain deployed draconian closures of most activities in communities where infection rates had been spreading exponentially. Others, such as Australia and New Zealand, closed down their societies and barricaded their borders to ensure no importation of the disease.

In the United Kingdom, the closure of society was implemented after some hesitancy. A scientific report based on epidemiological modelling presented the country's political leaders with a frightening worst-case scenario of up to half a million extra deaths caused by COVID-19. Without challenging the validity of these findings, the government made an about-turn in policy, shifting gear rapidly from a light-touch approach to a heave-handed alternative in which schools and university campuses were closed, people were told to stay home, not go to work unless they had to, and to restrict their trips from home for essential purposes such as once a day exercise and shopping for essentials. If they noticed symptoms in themselves that had been identified as typical of this new disease, such as fatigue, fever, a persistent cough, sore throat and loss of sense of taste or small, they should self-isolate for two weeks. Offices were closed, town and city centres were deserted, most high streets were shuttered, and public transportation systems were largely empty.

The public response was, by and large, positive, cooperative and constructive, certainly during the initial periods of "lockdowns" during the February to June period in 2020. This was true in many countries around the world. A few, such as Sweden, decided to persist with light-touch interventions and most people continued to go about their regular lives as normal. There were signs by the third month of restrictions on people's behaviour that patience was starting to wear thin, although fear responses that had been generated by many governments and public health authorities ultimately encouraged most people to behave as they were told. One side effect of this fear conditioning was that when societies did start to open up again during summer in 2020, many people remained too scared to venture out. Even the news media enjoined in a degree of complicity as purveyors of fear messages (Dodsworth, 2021).

As scientists forecast, despite its importance to the economy and to the psychological health of the population, coming out of lockdown and re-opening society posed the continued risk that, in doing so, the virus would once again spread widely and push up COVID-related hospitalisations and deaths. In due course, the prediction by senior medical and scientific experts that it would probably be necessary to re-introduce fresh waves of restrictions on public behaviour in the United Kingdom, including further lockdowns in different parts of the United Kingdom, as a "second wave" of COVID-19 occurred during the winter months of 2020 and into 2021.

During this time, however, hope was offered by the early development and regulatory approval of vaccines for COVID-19. Vaccination offered uncertain protection. They might protect against getting seriously ill, but not against getting infected and being able to spread it to others. These new vaccines were also found to be generally safe with minimal side effects for most people. A few, however, might experience serious side effects. Once vaccinated, everyone needed to understand that protection against the virus was not instantaneous but took time to take effect perhaps two to four weeks after inoculation. The issue was further complicated when reports appeared of new variants of the virus having emerged against which existing vaccines might or might not provide protection. In some instances, reports also indicated that new variants might be more infectious than the old ones.

Amidst this confusion, political leaders sowed further uncertainty by misrepresenting scientific understanding about these different features of the virus and the symptoms it could cause. One acute illustration of this point occurred in a briefing led by the United Kingdom's Prime Minister, Boris Johnson, on 22nd January 2021 when he stated that the new variant first detected in Kent, England, could kill up to 30% more people (Stewart et al., 2021). Yet, if he had studied research from his scientific advisors on this issue, he would have learned that the scientific evidence did not offer conclusive proof that the virus was more deadly to this extent. In fact, it collated data from several studies that had investigated non-representative samples of patients and deaths from different hospital locations with somewhat varying results. While all these studies generally pointed towards an indication that the new variant was somewhat more infectious than the old, it was too soon to know for sure that it could cause significantly more deaths.

The scientific advisers themselves were more circumspect in their conclusions drawn from this research (BBC News, 2021). They argued for continued and comprehensive restrictions on public behaviour in the face of this new virus which did seem to be driving the second wave of infections, but also called for much more evidence before firm conclusions could be reached about whether this new virus was a more serious killer as inferred by the prime minister's statement about it. Indeed, some of the most senior scientific and medical advisers tried to quell public fears by dampening down what the prime minister had said.

Psychology and Understanding Behavioural Compliance during the Pandemic

The biggest concern about the new coronavirus, SARS-CoV-2, was not its ability to kill lots of people, but the fact that it was infectious enough to be caught by many and although only a few would get really ill, they would still amount to a large number of people. The numbers of seriously ill could have the potential to overwhelm many national health systems. To make matters worse, of course, the fact that this was a new virus meant that there were many unknowns in terms of how to treat it. Further, there was no vaccine available to protect people from catching it. This meant, as experience with pandemics over many decades had shown, that in the absence of pharmaceutical treatments, NPIs would need to be deployed to bring the virus under control.

NPIs amounted mostly to behavioural interventions. Members of the public would be invited and encouraged to adopt specific personal hygiene practices such as washing their hands more than they would normally and trying to avoid interacting with other people in settings where there was a greater risk of becoming personally infected if in close contact with an already infected person.

Historical evidence, grounded in scientific analysis, dating back 100 years showed that getting people to adjust or change some of their usual behaviours could be effective in dealing with the spread of new infectious diseases (Cole, 2020). For instance, getting people to avoid going to places and spaces where there are crowds or large numbers of other people and spaces where they spend extended periods in the company of strangers can help to avoid the spread of a new virus. Closing down some spaces, such as schools or events where mass gatherings occur, might prove inconvenient to some and unpopular to many, but can also be effective. Also important is getting people to become aware of the most common symptoms caused by a new viral infection and to place themselves in quarantine for a specified time period if they find they are experiencing these symptoms themselves.

The scientific case for placing an entire region or country under draconian restrictions could readily be made on the basis of extant evidence. As we have seen, research into the Spanish flu pandemic 100 years before COVID had shown quite clearly that the timings of initiating lockdowns or other extreme restrictions and of their relaxation were critical not only to getting a current wave of infections under control but also to minimising the likelihood or even more damaging second and third waves (Bootsma & Ferguson, 2007).

Mathematical modelling with the novel coronavirus pandemic in different parts of the world confirmed historical data about the effectiveness of NPIs. Evidence also revealed that NPIs could vary in their effectiveness independently of the timings of their deployment (Block et al., 2020; Han et al., 2020; Ngonghala et al., 2020).

The challenge for governments when confronted with a major health crisis such as COVID-19 was to use the right tactics to command public compliance with any strategy reliant on NPIs. This required clear messaging about the risks of a virus and about the kinds of interventions that will be effective in protecting everyone from it. It also requires acknowledgement that to be effective, NPIs need to reach deep into people's lives and require that they put their normal, everyday activities on hold. Epidemiological modelling predicted that if certain interventions were deployed by governments, they would restrict public behaviour and this would in turn curtail transmission of the virus. The latter presumption about public behaviour was dependent upon whether people chose always to comply. Understanding whether they did or not and why they chose how to behave is a matter not addressed by epidemiological modellers, but these are questions studied by psychologists.

The Importance of Psychological Modelling

In 2020, COVID-19 pandemic lockdown scenario, nearly all national governments around the world sought to change public behaviour. Not all governments used the same interventions. When different governments did adopt a specific type of interventions, for example, the closure of schools, they did not all deploy an intervention in the same way. Another major characteristic of "lockdowns" or other forms of extensive behaviour restriction was that governments sought to change not one behaviour but many, all at the same time. In fact, governments frequently sought to persuade their people to put virtually all aspects of their normal lives on hold for an indefinite period. This might include not leaving home unless really necessary, not going to work, not seeing family and friends. For self-employed people, these restrictions often meant closing down their business operations. For everybody, it meant that most retail outlets were closed along with other important services such as hairdressers. Only essential outlets remained open, for example, those that provided food and everyday household, especially hygiene, products. Even then, there might be restricted times when specific categories of consumers were allowed inside specific retail outlets. There might also be long queues waiting to gain entry and temporary product supply shortages as some consumers "binge bought" specific product lines for personal stockpiling purposes. The collateral effects of pandemic-related behavioural restrictions are addressed in a separate volume (Gunter, 2022; *Psychological Impact of Behaviour Restrictions during the Pandemic: Lessons from COVID-19*). The present volume focuses on the psychology of public compliance with behaviour restrictions.

Health services such as dentists, optometrists and physiotherapists were suspended and most general practitioner appointments were available on a remote basis only. The catering and hospitality sectors were closed down except for home delivery and takeaway services. Culture, entertainment, leisure and sports venues and events were also closed down. People were told to avoid using public transport and making long journeys. Overseas holidays were also suspended.

It was important to model how all this could be achieved and virtually overnight. It was also important to model how such a lockdown could be sustained. There were hardships – financial and psychological – caused by the lockdown. These would represent disincentives to comply for very long. In addition, people would need to believe that the "cure" would work and was working. In addition, it would be necessary to model how everybody could be moved out of lockdown. As we saw in the last chapter, the epidemiological modelling failed to provide relevant guidance for a safe and strategic release from lockdown. Much the same could be said about the government's psychological modelling.

Early Evidence of Public Reactions

As the pandemic evolved over time, it might have been expected that the nature of people's reactions to it would also evolve. In the early days, there was a great deal of uncertainty about the new virus among the medical and scientific communities and among political leaders. It should not therefore be surprising if this uncertainty was not also present among people in general. Such uncertainty can make people more acutely aware of potential risks for themselves and others close to them and perhaps also at least a little afraid. For some sensitive personalities, these reactions might have been severe to a point of being debilitating. In the absence of vaccines, governments around the world relied instead upon NPIs to control the pandemic as COVID-19 cases mounted in their populations.

Research conducted even quite early in the 2020/2021 SARS-CoV-2 pandemic revealed commonalities in the reactions of people from different parts of the world, even when they lived in culturally disparate communities. However, what also emerged from some research is that early population to population differences in reactions to COVID-19 could be accounted for by the stage the pandemic had reached in specific parts of the world.

A comparison of the responses of people living in Hong Kong and the United Kingdom in the spring of 2020 confirmed this observation. Survey soundings were taken in Hong Kong between 24th January and 13th February 2020 and in the United Kingdom on 17th–18th March 2020. In Hong Kong, the disease was already established and, in the United Kingdom, it was also, but before the national lockdown many people were still unsure about how serious the full impact of the disease was likely to get (Bowman et al., 2021).

People in Hong Kong displayed much more widespread concern (97%) about the severity of the disease than did people in the United Kingdom (20%). More people in Hong Kong (60%) compared with the United Kingdom (47%) reported some degree of anxiety about this new coronavirus. There was widespread awareness in both locations, no the dates of these surveys, that the new virus was airborne. Adoption of preventive behaviours was more widespread in Hong Kong than in the United Kingdom, especially face mask wearing (99% vs. 3%). In Hong Kong, various preventive measures had already been adopted by virtually everybody whereas in the United Kingdom they were more likely to have been adopted by those individuals who perceived transmission through the air as "easy" and the effects of the disease as "severe".

As noted earlier, four psychological models are examined in this book in relation to the study of people's behavioural compliance with COVID-19 restrictions. These models are nudge theory, the theory of planned behaviour, the Compatibility-Opportunity-Motivation-Behaviour model and social identity/group processes theory. Each of these theories is introduced briefly here and then each is discussed in more detail in the following four chapters.

Nudge Theory

Nudge theory proposed that people's behaviour could be changed through subtle influences implemented in their surrounding environment. Such influences might be verbal or non-verbal in nature. They might signal specific behavioural choices to people or encourage them to take their behaviour in a specific direction. Nudges would sometimes present behavioural options for individuals to choose between and then might encourage them to choose one over the other (Thaler & Sunstein, 2009).

Some nudging is achieved through messages that present behavioural options to people with further information about potential outcomes. These options can then be weighed in the balance and individuals can choose which way to go (Parkinson et al., 2014; Saghai, 2013). Hence, there may be an element of persuasion in nudging, but it tends to be subtly deployed.

There are other occasions when messages are presented to audiences through the media about outcome probabilities that are also attached to risk estimates. In the context of the COVID-19 pandemic, for instance, much early media attention to infection rates gave the impression that the health crisis was getting worse. Further emphasis on mortality rates linked to COVID-19, though in reality rare, gave the impression that they were frequently occurring. Hence, even though the statistical probability of an individual dying of COVID-19 was low, the attention given to death rates created a subjective impression among many people that it was common-place. This psychological phenomenon was described by psychologists as the "availability heuristic". This concept posited that when people make decisions about how to behave, they consider cost and benefit probabilities linked to different options. If one outcome has been given more attention than the other, they may be more likely to allow that one to influence their eventual behaviour the most (Chapman, 1967; Tversky & Kahneman, 1973, 1979).

Group Processes and Social Identity Model

Maintaining the public's commitment to draconian restrictions on their normal freedom of movement can be reinforced by creating a sense of collective responsibility. Put simply, this means that everyone in a community or group or society must put aside selfish impulses and wishes and act instead in everyone's best interests. This does not mean that everyone is expected to act like mindless automatons or communities driven by a narrow groupthink mentality. It is important always that collectives consider the reasons or explanations for courses of action they are being invited to take.

During the pandemic, people were regularly reminded of the risks posed by the new virus and also by not following their government's advice. This meant that a degree of trust in government was necessary and if that was damaged, so too could the public's willingness to behave according to the new pandemic rulebook. When it came to assessments of risk from the coronavirus, each individual took a personal view of their own risk. This represented a factor that influenced their decision making about any miti-gating steps they might take to safeguard themselves. At the level of the collective, however, there must ultimately be a consensus position reached with everyone acting together in unison or at least in some sort of harmony. Individuals might have perceived their personal risk from COVID-19 as being modest but if they then were concerned about the risks to wider social groups, especially groups to which they belonged, their willingness to comply with behavioural restrictions persisted over time (Franzen & Wohner, 2021). Keeping things this way, however, depends in part on the behaviour of others as well as self and then upon how the behaviour of others is perceived. In more general terms, research showed that adherence to a collectivistic over an individualistic worldview, where the greater social good was prioritised over self-interest showed more persistent compliance with pandemic-related behavioural restrictions (Siegrist & Bearth, 2021).

By becoming part of a collective that works together, individuals can gain psychological sustenance that not only helps to keep them on track with restrictions and guidelines about how they should behave, but also empowers them in a way in which they feel they have more control over an uncertain situation and this can reduce anxiety responses and keep them generally in a healthier state (Haslam et al., 2018).

A social identity model was therefore recommended by some psychologists on the grounds that this would create the right mindset to reinforce behaviour encouraged by the slogan, "we are all in this together". Social identity theory was devised as a model for analysis of how human behaviour could be influenced by individuals' sense that they belonged to specific social groups (Tajfel, 1974; Tajfel & Turner, 1979). In identifying with a group, individuals developed a sense of "social identity" that sat alongside their sense of "personal identity" (Tajfel & Turner, 2004; Turner et al., 1987).

Evidence emerged that social identity can mediate people's responses to government interventions during crises such as a pandemic. Governments' responses to a pandemic can create new groupings of people defined by their relative risks of infection or of becoming seriously ill once infected. Other divisions among populations can also emerge based on people's reactions to different kinds of government advice, for example, in relation to wearing face masks, observing physical distancing and getting vaccinated. Sometimes these divisions emerge from pre-existing "tribes" or communities, and sometimes they emerge for the first time during a pandemic (Templeton et al., 2020). Later in this book, further evidence will be provided to demonstrate further how social identity and group processes were psychological variables that could be used to drive behavioural compliance.

Theory of Planned Behaviour

Another popular theoretical framework for analysing and predicting behaviour change has been the theory of planned behaviour. This theory grew out of an earlier iteration known as the theory of reasoned action. Essentially, this theory has identified that a person's overt behaviour choices are influenced by internal cognitive constructs such as their beliefs about and attitudes towards that behaviour (Ajzen, 1991). A pandemic example might be the willingness to get vaccinated. This action is more likely to occur when an individual believes that it will have more benefits than costs (belief) and feels that it is the right thing to do (positive attitude).

This notion was articulated in the theory of reasoned action but when it was empirically tested, the emergent evidence showed that this framework sometimes predicted behaviour outcomes accurately, but not always. One reason why it sometimes failed to explain behaviour choices was that there were other cognitive factors that were important to people's behaviour choices. They needed to see that other people were adopting a specific behavioural option. This factor was called "subjective norm". Such behaviour reinforced the individual to make the same choice under pressure of social conformity and because of their perception that if other people were making a specific behaviour choice, perhaps they should do the same.

Another factor then emerged that seemed to be even more crucial to the individual's eventual behaviour choice. This was the perception on the part of the individual that they were able to enact that specific behaviour. This factor was called "perceived behavioural control". Once again, in the pandemic context, the willingness of some groups of people, such as teenagers, to get vaccinated, was weakened when they witnessed other teenagers refusing to do so. Furthermore, when evidence emerged that there were potentially harmful side effects from vaccines and that these were most likely to affect young people, this knowledge also discouraged their compliance with requests from authorities to get vaccinated. Then, if the nearest vaccination centre was a long way off and there was no easy way of getting to it, an individual might not get vaccinated simply because the behaviour was beyond their resources or ability (see Ajzen & Fishbein, 1980).

COM-B Model

Psychologists that study behaviour change and the efficacy of nudging and overt persuasive techniques operating through series of internal attitudes and beliefs have found that other predictors of behaviour choice exist. Both nudging and reasoning can be effective in shaping behaviour choices – but not always. On some occasions, understanding has to be sought that goes beyond the explanatory limits of these theoretical frameworks. Both of these models restrict their theories to specific sets of variables that underpin intentions or motives to perform specific behaviours. There may be occasions and settings when these methods are not enough to achieve the desired behavioural responses.

Conducting a wider scan of psychological literature about behaviour conditioning and change, psychologists have discovered other theoretical constructs that can have explanatory or predictive potential with behaviour. It might therefore be logical to adopt a more pragmatic approach to a theory about behaviour and the design of behaviour change programmes to manipulate the public's actions. New concepts were introduced alongside old ones. The new model included behaviour change as its eventual outcome and included a concept of "motivation" as a key driver of change. Prior to that, it was deemed to be important to assess the ability of an individual to embrace and enact change in a specific setting or context and this idea was embodied in the construct of "capability". Then, the specific situation in which behaviour change was required to occur needed to provide the necessary "opportunity" for an individual to adopt a specific behaviour pattern (Bish & Michie, 2010).

This framework was called the capability-opportunity-motivation-behaviour (COM-B) model. It could be applied to situations in which there were potentially a number of distinct interventions in an individual's circumstances that could influence their behaviour choices. The efficacy of these might vary from situation to situation and with the type of behaviour being influenced. It might also vary or be mediated by the internal characteristics of the individual such as their personality profile. In devising an analytical model that needed to embrace or represent a wide range of variables, it might also have to knit together a number of distinct theories of human behaviour (Michie et al., 2005). Some of these theories might concern specific types of behaviour and not others. Hence, the eventual choices of constructs to include and measure in an analysis would be driven by relevant empirical evidence and knowledge of the indigenous strengths and weaknesses of different theories. In other words, the overall approach was a pragmatic one rather than being rigidly tied to one specific theoretical dogma (Aunger et al., 2016; Michie et al., 2009).

This book will examine what was learned about the willingness of entire national populations to accept and comply with often draconian restrictions by their governments during 2020–2021 when a new coronavirus pandemic swept across the globe. People's normal everyday lives were upended as they were advised or even instructed to stay home and to venture out only occasionally for a narrow range of reasons and while following stringent behavioural protocols. Although many different scientific disciplines were invited to assist governments to advise on how drastic interventions could be implemented, understanding how people reacted cognitively, emotionally and behaviourally to these unprecedented circumstances falls squarely within the domain of psychology.

Psychologists can call upon a vast body of research accumulated over many decades to formulate models of human behaviour that can indicate if not predict how people of different kinds will respond when they are told to suspend normal life. In the context of the novel coronavirus pandemic, four behavioural models in particular were consulted the most. These are introduced above and will now be reviewed in more depth in the chapter that follows. As the book progresses, the reader will also be introduced to a vast body of new research that emerged during the 2020–2021 period that investigated the efficacy of these models in guiding effective pandemic intervention strategies.

References

Ajzen, I. (1991). The theory of planned behavior. *Organizational Behavior and Human Decision Processes, 50*(2), 179–211.

Ajzen, I., & Fishbein, M. (1980). *Understanding Attitudes and Predicting Social Behavior*. Englewood-Cliffs, NJ: Prentice-Hall.

Arnot, M. et al. (2020). How evolutionary behavioural sciences can help us understand behaviour in a pandemic. *Evolution, Medicine, and Public Health*, 2020(1), 264–278. doi: 10.1093/emph/eoaa038

Aunger, R., Greenland, K., Ploubidis, G., Schmidt, W., Oxford, J., & Curtis, V. (2016). The determinants of reported personal and household hygiene behaviour: A multi-country study. *PLoS One*, 11(8), e0159551.

Barry, J. M. (2004). *The Great Influenza: The Story of the Greatest Plague in History*. New York, NY: Viking Press.

Bavel, J. J. V. et al. (2020). Using social and behavioural science to support COVID-19 pandemic response. *Nature and Human Behaviour*, 4(5), 460–471. doi: 10.1038/s41562-020-0884-z

BBC News. (2021, 23rd January). Covid: 'Ore deadly' UK variant claim played down by scientists. Retrieved from: https://www.bbc.co.uk/news/uk-55779171

Bish, A., & Michie, S. (2010). Demographic and attitudinal determinants of protective behaviours during a pandemic: A review. *British Journal of Health Psychology*, 15(4), 797–824.

Block, P., Hoffman, M., Raabe, I. J., Dowd, J. B., Rahal, C., Kashyap, R., & Mills, M. C. (2020). Social network-based distancing strategies to flatten the COVID-19 curve in a post-lockdown world. *Nature Human Behaviour*, 4(6), 588–596.

Bonell, C. et al. (2020). Harnessing behavioural science in public health campaigns to maintain 'social distancing' in response to the COVID-19 pandemic: Key principles. *Journal of Epidemiology & Community Health*, 74(8), 617–619. doi: 10.1136/jech-2020-214290

Bootsma, M. C. J., & Ferguson, N.M. (2007). The effect of public health measures on the 1918 influenza pandemic in U.S. cities. *Proceedings of the National Academy of Science, USA*, 104(18), 7588–7593.

Bowman, L., Kwok, K. O., Redd, R., Yi, Y., Ward, H., Wei, W. I., Atchison, C., & Wong, S. Y. (2021). Comparing public perceptions and preventive behaviors during the early phase of the COVID-19 pandemic in Hong Kong and the United Kingdom: Cross-sectional survey study. *Journal of Medicine and Internet Research*, 23(3), e23231. https://doi.org/10.2196/23231

Brilliant, L. (2006, February). My wish: Help me stop pandemics. TED Talks. Retrieved from: https://www.ted.com/talks/larry_brilliant_my_wish_help_me_stop_pandemics?language=en

Chapman, L. J. (1967). Illusory correlation in observational report. *Journal of Verbal Learning*, 6, 151–155.

Cole, J. (2020, 26th March). Coronavirus: Why changing human behaviour is the best defence in tackling the virus. *The Conversation*. Available at: https://theconversation.com/coronavirus-why-changing-human-behaviour-is-the-best-defence-in-tackling-the-virus-134500

Cook, A. R., Zhao, X., Chen, M. I. C., & Finkelstein, E. A. (2018). Public preferences for interventions to prevent emerging infectious disease threats: A discrete choice experiment. *BMJ Open*, 8(2), e017355. https://doi.org/10.1136/bmjopen-2017-017355

Dodsworth, L. (2021). *A State of Fear*. London, UK: Pinter & Martin Ltd.

FEMA (Federal Emergency Management Agency). (2019, 25th July). 2019 national threat and hazard identification and risk assessment (THIRA): Overview and methodology. US Department of Homeland Security. Retrieved from: www. hsdl.org

Ferguson, N. M., Laydon, D., Nedjati-Gilani, G., et al. (2020, 16th March). *Impact of non-pharmaceutical interventions (NPIs) to reduce COVID-19 mortality and healthcare demand*. Imperial College London. https://doi.org/10.25561/77482. Available at: https://spiral.imperial.ac.uk:8443/bitstream/10044/1/77482/14/2020-03-16-COVID19-Report-9.pdf

Flaxman, S., Mishra, S., Gandy, A. et al. (2020). Estimating the effects of non-pharmaceutical interventions on COVID-19 in Europe. *Nature, 584*, 257–261. https://doi.org/10.1038/s41586-020-2405-7

Franzen, A., & Wohner, F. (2021). Coronavirus risk perception and compliance with social distancing measures in a sample of young adults: Evidence from Switzerland. *PloS One*. Retrieved from: https://journals.plos.org/plosone/article?id=10.1371/journal.pone.0247447

Gunter, B. (2022). *Psychological Impact of Behaviour Restrictions during the Pandemic: Lessons from COVID-19*. Abingdpn, UK: Routledge.

Han, E., Tan, M. M. J., Turk, E., Sridhar, D., Leung, G. M., Shibuya, K., et al. (2020). Lessons learnt from easing COVID-19 restrictions: An analysis of countries and regions in Asia Pacific and Europe. *The Lancet, 396*(10261), 1525–1534.

Haslam, S. A., McMahon, C., Cruwys, T., Haslam, C., Jetten, J., & Steffens, N. K. (2018). Social cure, what social cure? The propensity to underestimate the importance of social factors for health. *Social Science & Medicine, 198*, 14–21.

Heneghan, C., & Jefferson, T. (2020, 9th April) COVID-19 deaths compared with "Swine Flu". The centre for Evidence-Based Medicine, University of Oxford, Available at: https://www.cebm.net/covid-19/covid-19-deaths-compared-with-swine-flu/

Henig, R. M. (2020, 9th April). Experts warned of a pandemic decades ago. Why weren't we ready? *National Geographic*. Retrieved from: https://www.nationalgeographic.co.uk/science-and-technology/2020/04/experts-warned-of-pandemic-decades-ago-why-werent-we-ready

Jeffery, K. T., & David, M. M. (2006). 1918 influenza: The mother of all pandemics. *Emerging Infectious Disease journal, 12*(1), 15–22.

Kalnins, I. (2006). The Spanish influenza of 1918 in St Louis, Missouri. *Public Health Nursing, 23*(5), 479–483.

Mackenzie, D. (2020). *COVID-19: The Pandemic That Never Should Have Happened and How to Stop the Next One*. London, UK: Little, Brown.

Markel, H., Lipman, H. B., Navarro, J. A., Sloan, A., Michalsen, J. R., Stern, A. M., & Cetron, M. S. (2007). Nonpharmaceutical interventions implemented by US cities during the 19818–1919 influenza pandemic. *Journal of the American Medical Association, 298*(6), 644–654.

McGrath, C. (2019, 25th October). Pandemic warning: Terrifying new report warns every country on Earth is at risk. *Express*. Retrieved from: https://www.express.co.uk/news/world/1195719/global-pandemic-ebola-epidemic-pathogen-disease-biological-warfare-latest-news-update

Menachery, V. D., Yount, B. L. Jr., Sims, A. C., Debbink, K., Agnihothram, S. S., Gralinski, L. E., Graham, R. L., Scobey, T., Plante, J. A., Royal, S. R., Swanstrom, J., Sheahan, T. P., Pickles, R. J., Corti, D., Randell, S. H., Lanzavecchia, A., Marasco, W. A., & Baric, R. S. (2016). SARS-like WIV1-CoV poised for human emergence. *Proceedings of the National Academy of Sciences of the United States of America, 113*(11), 3048–3053. https://doi.org/10.1073/pnas.1517719113

Michie, S. (2020). Behavioural, environmental, social and systems interventions against covid-19. *BMJ, 370.* https://doi.org/10.1136/bmj.m2982

Michie, S., Abraham, C., Whittington, C., McAteer, J., & Gupta, S. (2009). Effective techniques in healthy eating and physical activity interventions: A meta-regression. *Health Psychology, 28*(6), 690–701. https://doi.org/10.1037/a001 6136

Michie, S., & Johnston, M. (2012). Theories and techniques of behaviour change: Developing a cumulative science of behaviour change. *Health Psychology Review, 6,* 1–6.

Michie, S., Johnston, M., Abraham, C., Lawton, R., Parker, D., & Walker, A. (2005). "Psychological Theory" group. Making psychological theory useful for implementing evidence-based practice: A consensus approach. *BMJ: Quality and Safety, 14*(1), 26–33. https://doi.org/10.1136/qshc.2004.011155

Neville, F. G., Templeton, A., Smith, J. R., & Louis, W. R. (2021). Social norms, social identities and the COVID-19 pandemic: Theory and recommendations. *Social and Personality Psychology Compass, 15*(5), e12596. https://doi.org/1 0.1111/spc3.12596

Ngonghala, C. N., Iboi, E., Eikenberry, S., Scotch, M., MacIntyre, C. R., Bonds, M. H., & Gumel, A. B. (2020). Mathematical assessment of the impact of non-pharmaceutical interventions on curtailing the 2019 novel coronavirus. *Mathematical Biosciences, 325,* 108364. https://doi.org/10.1016/j.mbs.2020.1 08364

NHS (2009). Swine flu (H1N1). Retrieved from: https://www.nhs.uk/conditions/swine-flu/

Parkinson, J. A., Eccles, K. E., & Goodman, A. (2014). Positive impact by design: The Wales Centre for behaviour change. *Journal of Positive Psychology, 9*(6), 517–522.

Saghai, Y. (2013). Salvaging the concept of nudge. *Journal of Medical Ethics, 39*(8), 487–493.

Siegrist, M., & Bearth, A. (2021). Worldviews, trust and risk perceptions shape public acceptance of COVID-19 public health measures. *Proceedings of the National Academy of Sciences of the United States of America, 118*(24), e2100411118. https://doi.org/10.1073/pnas.2100411118

Stewart, H., Sample, J., & Davis, N. (2021, 23rd January). New UK Covid variant may be 30% more deadly, says Boris Johnson. *The Guardian.* Retrieved from: https://www.theguardian.com/world/2021/jan/22/new-uk-covid-variant-may-be-more-deadly-says-boris-johnson

Tajfel, H. (1974). Social identity and intergroup behaviour. *Social Science Information, 13*(2), 65–93.

Tajfel, H., & Turner, J. C. (1979). An integrative theory of inter-group conflict. In W. G. Austin, & S. Worchel (Eds.), *The Social Psychology of Inter-Group Relations* (pp. 33–47). Monterey, CA: Brooks/Cole.

Tajfel, H., & Turner, J. C. (2004). The social identity theory of intergroup behaviour. In J. T. Jost & J. Sidanius (Eds.), *Political Psychology: Key Readings* (pp. 276–293). Brighton, UK: Psychology Press.

Templeton, A., Guven, S. T., Hoerst, C., Vestergren, S., Davidson, L., Ballentyne, S., Madsen, H., & Choudhury, S. (2020). Inequalities and identity processes in crises: Recommendations for facilitating safe response to the COVID-19 pandemic. *British Journal of Social Psychology*, 59(3), 674–685. https://doi.org/1 0.1111/bjso.12400

Thaler, R., & Sunstein, C. (2009) *Nudge: Improving Decisions about Health, Wealth and Happiness*. Oxford, UK: Blackwell.

Turner, J. C. (1975). Social comparison and social identity: Some prospects for intergroup behaviour. *European Journal of Social Psychology*, 5, 5–34.

Turner, J. C., Hogg, M., Oakes, P., Reicher, S., & Wetherell, M. (1987). *Rediscovering the Social Group: A Self-Categorisation Theory*. Oxford, UK: Basil Blackwell.

Tversky, A., & Kahneman, D. (1973). Availability: A heuristic for judging frequency and probability. *Cognitive Psychology*, 5(2), 207–232.

Tversky, A., & Kahneman, D. (1979). Prospect theory: An analysis of decision under risk. *Econometrica*, 47(2), 263–291.

World Health Organization. (2020). Listing of WHO's responses to COVID-19. (Originally compiled 29th June 2020; updated on 28th December 2020.) Retrieved from: https://www.who.int/news/item/29-06-2020-covidtimeline

Yong, E. (2018, July/August). The next plague is coming. Is America ready? *The Atlantic*. Retrieved from: https://www.theatlantic.com/magazine/archive/2018/ 07/when-the-next-plague-hits/561734/

Chapter 2

Psychological Modelling: Nudging Behaviour Change

Governments around the world took much advice from scientists and these scientists came from many different disciplines. As the pandemic surfaced, epidemiologists produced projections of the spread of the new virus among specific populations and also modelled the likely impact of specific non-pharmaceutical interventions (NPIs) in terms of controlling infection rates. These macro-societal-level analyses were often based on assumptions about the predicted impacts of specific sets of intervention variables that had not all been well-defined in operational terms and whose individual effects had not yet been validated. Moreover, these interventions were sometimes treated as having equivalent weights of impact despite not having been implemented the same way in different countries or in different regions within the same country (Ferguson et al., 2020). The extent to which people's behaviour patterns could change and these changes then accurately measured, following the implementation of NPIs, posed challenges and raised questions that the epidemiology was ill-equipped to answer.

Epidemiologists advised governments about the efficacy of specific NPIs in halting the spread of the virus. Yet, the eventual effectiveness of these measures depended upon the extent to which the public complied behaviourally with these interventions. The efficacy of the modelling depended on the presence of compelling empirical verification of the impacts of specific interventions on specific public behaviours and the relevance of the latter to minimising virus transmission.

This volume will not focus on macro-level epidemiology. Some of the initial epidemiological modelling failed to consider the impact of specific interventions at a sufficient level of granularity. They tended to measure the application of these interventions in a binary fashion when linear measures would have provided much more analytical and predictive power. There is an additional level of analysis which is particularly important, however, when trying to understand behavioural compliance with government or public health restrictions and this derives from psychology modelling of public behavioural choices. This means that we need to know how people can be

DOI: 10.4324/9781003274308-2

persuaded to "do as they are told" in terms of performing new behaviours to protect themselves against infection and withdrawing from n activities that present virus transmission risks.

Whether individuals will be persuaded to adopt new behaviours and suspend old ones is a question that requires some understanding of people's psychology. What do people think and feel about the changes being imposed on their lives during lockdown? Do they like or dislike them? Do they regard compliance as reasonable or feasible in the context of their own lives? Do they trust not only the messages they receive but also the sources of those messages, that is, the politicians and scientists? These are all questions that need to be answered to understand how specific non-pharmacological interventions will command public cooperation in the short term as well as how much they might be tolerated in the longer term should that become necessary.

In addition to initial acceptance and compliance, it is important to know which interventions within a pandemic lockdown will be easiest to gain compliance and which will people tolerate for the longest. With many lockdown interventions, there will be further questions about the harms they might cause to people financially and psychologically in the longer term and even in the short term. If the side effects are unpalatable and potentially more harmful than the virus could be if infected, both for the individual and for society, this fact would necessitate a re-think about how to tackle the pandemic.

Nudging and Behaviour Control

A popular branch of "behaviour-change" psychology that has been used by governments across a wide span of public policy decisions has been popularly referred to as "nudge theory". It is concerned with subtle environmental manipulations of public perceptions to gently push their behaviour in a desired direction. In doing this, the recipients are not "persuaded" to change their minds so much as encouraged to shift their behaviour in a way over which they take personal ownership. This sense of ownership derives from the frequent use of "invitations" to people to make their own risk assessments of different choices on the basis of specific experiences they have or information with which they have been supplied.

Nudge theory cuts across a number of social sciences but essentially comprises a psychological theory of how people's decisions can be influenced by subtle manipulations of conditions in their environment. The concept of nudging was popularised by two American academics, Richard Thaler and Cass Sunstein in their book published in 2008, titled *Nudge: Improving Decisions about Health, Wealth and Happiness*. The fundamental premise of this work was that it is possible to change people's behaviours through subtle influences that work on the basis of drawing their attention to behavioural options and gently pushing them towards the option that influencers want them to adopt. This approach entails behaviour change without coercion and philosophically has been labelled as libertarian paternalism (Thaler & Sunstein, 2009).

When creating the conditions to encourage people to change their behaviour or to adopt a new behaviour, a decision-making framework is constructed in which choice options are outlined with information attached to encourage and inform rational decision making. It is possible to "nudge" people towards the preferred behaviour by constructing persuasive messages that encourage cognitive information processing that leads them in this direction and leaves them believing that the choice was all their own idea (Parkinson et al., 2014; Saghai, 2013). Hence, persuasive messages are designed to trigger thoughts about the options that encourage one option to be selected over the other(s). This process is shaped by the choice architecture of a persuasive campaign or programme of change.

Nudge theory uses environmental and psychological cues to prompt people to change their behaviour. The aim here is to change behaviour not through direct persuasive argumentation or through autocratic commands, but in a more subtle way by signposting directions for behaviour within different settings using physical cues. Nudge approaches centre on introducing new elements and features into the "architecture" of specific environments. These features might include signage asking people to do certain things, attention-drawing stimuli that pull people in a particular direction and physical changes to routes through specific environmental settings. Retail outlets might introduce scents (i.e., the smell of freshly baked bread) near the shelves or counter where baked products are being sold. Markings might be painted onto roads that are gradually positioned closer and closer together giving the impression of increased speed when driving over them, to encourage drivers to slow down at accident blackspots. They might comprise painted targets on urinals that encourage users to be more accurate in hitting the target rather than the surrounding floor or wall.

This approach to behaviour change has been applied in numerous fields but has especially widely used in the public health sphere. It is no surprise that "nudging" had been used by the British Conservative government for many years before the SARS-CoV-2 pandemic hit the country (Rigby, 2020).

Former Prime Minister David Cameron set up the Behavioural Insights Team (also known colloquially as the "nudge unit") in 2010 to inform government decision making on policy matters designed to produce public behaviour changes. Nudge theory has also been used by other governments around the world and major international bodies such as the United Nations, World Bank and European Commission.

Nudge theory as used by the British government was influenced by the writings of Richard Thaler and Cass Sunstein who wrote a best-selling book on the subject, *Nudge: Improving Decisions about Health, Wealth and Happiness*. Nudging was conceived as a system for using "priming techniques" or prompts to encourage people to change their behaviours. The approach was concerned less with simply telling people in a paternalistic way that they needed to change and instead presented people with options to choose from (Thaler & Sunstein, 2009).

Psychological Origins of "Nudging"

The "nudge" concept did not originate with Thaler and Sunstein, however. It evolved from the work of two Nobel Prize winning psychologists, also widely recognised as founding fathers of behavioural economics, Amos Tversky and Daniel Kahneman. They were interested in the way that people think about risk and the frequencies with which events occur. One central concept they discussed was the "availability heuristic". This idea posited that whenever we need to make decisions between options concerning our behaviour or when judging phenomena, we make personal calculations that draw primarily on examples that most readily spring to mind. For example, if two events occur together on a few occasions, we might be tempted to believe that they always occur together when in fact they rarely do (Chapman, 1967).

Tversky and Kahneman (1973) found that if people were asked to think of words beginning with the letter "k" or words that had "k" as their third letter, they were more readily able to think of the former than the latter. They then also believed that words beginning in a "k" were more commonplace than words with "k" as their third letter. There was no statistical evidence to prove that this assumption was correct. Nevertheless, this belief was powerfully expressed, according to the researchers, because some words were more "available" in a cognitive sense to the people making these judgements.

The Availability Heuristic

What seems to happen when people make judgements about the commonality of specific objects, events, issues or topics is that estimated frequencies rely on relevant examples that can be most readily recalled in that moment. If there are two sets of events that in real terms occurred equally often, but where one set stands out from the rest, the most prominent set will be better recalled and those recalling these events will also believe they tend to occur more often (when they do not).

In an experiment designed to demonstrate this phenomenon, Tversky and Kahneman (1973) presented participants with the names of 19 famous women and 20 less famous men or of 19 famous men and 20 less famous women. Subsequently, the participants were invited to recall as many names as possible and estimate whether there were more women or more men named in the list. The celebrities' names were recalled most often from both lists and the gender associated with the most famous names was thought to occur more frequently than the gender linked to the less famous names. Prominence via celebrity status made those names stand out more during learning and this rendered them more memorable later on. This memory advantage also led those taking part in the experiment to make frequency judgement errors about how often different types of names were re-presented.

These "availability" effects on our judgements about how often specific events occur and about any risks to us that might be associated with them are not restricted to the laboratory. They can also occur in everyday life as a result of specific life experiences. Despite its claims to objectivity, news coverage tends to prefer to report unusual rather than regular events. The dependence of many people on the news, especially on television, where events can be vividly displayed, might lead some frequency or probability judgements about events to be skewed by news reports. Hence, while deaths from shark attacks were found to be more frequently reported in the news than deaths from parts falling off aeroplanes, in actual statistical terms people were more likely to be killed by falling bits from planes (Read, 1995).

Other research has shown that people's estimates of risks from crime and violence can be shaped by their television viewing experiences. This effect can result from exposure not just to news broadcasts but also to fictional drama programmes (Gunter, 1987; Riddle, 2010). The viewing of televised depictions of specific acts of violence and themes covering police corruption and criminality triggered heightened beliefs about the frequency of such incidents in the real world (Riddle, 2010).

Despite the rarity of such incidents, their "availability" in memory for people exposed to vivid television portrayals of these events rendered them more reality available when real-world estimates of how often such events occurred were tested. Further evidence has shown, however, that these "availability" or prompting effects of perceived frequencies of events might be short-lived. If they represent new information about a topic and assume that the information is perceived as credible, it might exert an initial impact on public perceptions of event frequencies, but this effect can dissipate after a week or two (Sjöberg & Engelberg, 2010).

What we do need to be mindful of in this case is whether the "new" information is subsequently repeated to a point where it comes to be seen as legitimate and accurate and is deeply conditioned in people's minds over time. Where the potential priming of risks from SARS-CoV-2 via daily and incessant news coverage was concerned, constant reminders of death risk could become highly resilient. As we will see when examining data for public opinion about release of COVID-19 lockdown restrictions, many people remained cautious and even fearful about loosening of government-imposed interventions that were designed to protect them from a clear and present danger.

Losses versus Benefits

Another related concept is "loss aversion". This phenomenon was discovered by psychologists many years ago. What this idea refers to is the finding that when we are required to make judgements, our decisions can be influenced more powerfully by the losses we calculate to follow on from our behaviour than by the perceived personal benefits of it (Tversky & Kahneman, 1979). It seems we are more willing to take risks to avoid loss than to win benefits or awards, even when the magnitude of the loss does not exceed the size of the gain (Tversky & Kahneman, 1979). The way losses and gains are framed when individuals are confronted with taking critical decisions can make a significant difference in risk-taking (Haigh & List, 2005; Segev et al., 2015).

Heuristic-Systematic Model of Persuasion

The heuristic-systematic model offers a similar perspective on how people can be persuaded to change their attitudes and ultimately their behaviour to the one provided by the elaboration-likelihood model. The latter differentiated between central and peripheral processing of persuasion messages. This model distinguishes between systematic processing of information in a message and heuristic processing.

This dual process system was explained by Daniel Kahneman, who distinguished between two systems for processing information that he called "fast" and "slow". Fast processing tended to be more automatic, while slow processing was more reflective. In one situation (System 1), individuals reached quick judgements that could be influenced by external factors such as the characteristics of messages from agencies trying to trigger specific behavioural responses. In the other (System 2), the individual weighed up messages and considered the meaning and relevance of their contents, deciding on the basis of rational judgement whether or not to take on board what was being said. Fast processing has also been described as based on the use of heuristic devices and slow processing tends to be more reflective and systematic in the decision making it encourages (Kahneman, 2003).

Slow processing occupied more cognitive capacity and required more time and mental resources to be performed effectively. Under pressure of time and/or when attentional demands were experienced from different directions, fast-processing would take over and more superficial judgements about messages were usually made. Fast-processing takes shortcuts and this can lead to poor decisions being made. There are behaviour patterns, for instance, that have been repeated so often that they become habitual. This means that we continue to behave in a tried-and-tested way without giving the matter much thought. Often, this process may not cause problems for us, but if our behaviours are no longer fit for purpose in a given setting because historical conditions have changed, our reluctance to focus enough to adapt can result in action that will no longer serve us well. With deeply conditioned habits, significant environmental changes are often needed to trigger a change in us (Campbell-Arvai et al., 2014; Thaler & Sunstein, 2009).

One illustration of this behaviour might be that we drive to work taking the same route every day and eventually do so without even being consciously aware of the journey. Then an accident occurs causing a road blockage necessitating a change in direction. This might cause us then to devise contingency routes for the future in the event that similar incidents occur at different points along the usual route.

Similarly, if we shop in the same supermarket several times a week, we develop a mental map of the layout of the store which enables us to know instantly where to go to get to specific product ranges. Then, one day we enter the store to find that a new manager has changed the layout and nothing is where it used to be. Now we have to devote mental effort to find the items we normally buy making the experience more cognitively taxing than it usually is. As such we might miss the special offers on products we would not usually buy, but might when they are offered at premium prices. Yet, at the same time, by placing products we would not usually buy on shelves where we routinely expect to find something else might also encourage us to buy those products because for once they have grabbed our attention. This could have positive benefits if healthy fruits and vegetables are positioned where junk foods used to be and we would generally head for the processed products that are less nutritious and good for our health.

Nudge approaches are used in settings where System 1 decision making is likely to be triggered in order to counter rash choices. The influencer makes the initial judgement about the direction in which behaviour should change and then provides cues or hints designed to push people towards that preferred behaviour. One example of this type of nudging derives from a diet change context. In encouraging people to eat healthy foods while steering them away from junk foods, stores were invited to place healthy food options near the checkout counter where they were both visible and placed in a setting in which customers were often required to stand in line and therefore had an opportunity to notice these foods. The proximity to the checkouts where customers paid for their goods also created a mindset in that moment of paying for purchases which might also encourage purchase of healthy food options just before leaving the store (Kroese et al., 2016).

In systematic processing, we assess the value and veracity of the information in a persuasion message to determine whether we believe it to be accurate, authentic, reliable, relevant and truthful. In performing this process, we might draw upon what we already know about the topic communicated in the message as well as about the message source. We might then weigh up the information in the message against that derived from other sources. Our decisions about whether to maintain or change our current attitudes or formulate new attitudes based on the information received in the message follow from these careful deliberations (Chen & Chaiken, 1999).

Systematic processing, such as central processing, requires a lot of effort and we cannot always be bothered to give an issue that level of consideration before making our minds up about it. We seek shortcuts to reaching a decision about whether our current attitude is robust or should be changed. This is where heuristics come into play. One application of heuristics is to consider what we know about other people's attitudes and behaviours. If the message asks us to think about a topic in a certain way or to behave in a certain fashion, and we can see that others do likewise, we might decide to follow the consensus. We presume that if other people look favourably on an object or specific issue-position, then we could do worse than following their lead. We might instead turn our attention to the advice or actions of trusted others, such as experts or authorities, or perhaps people we know well.

If an advertisement recommends a furniture supplier with which we are personally unfamiliar, but someone we know has given them a recommendation, then we might be more ready to accept what the commercial says and be more ready to use that supplier ourselves.

A heuristic approach might save mental effort, but it does not always lead us to make the best judgements. One of the ways in which this can happen is when someone tries to persuade us to change our behaviour, promising some personal advantage or benefit from doing so. They might also indicate that by not adopting the behaviour they recommend, there could be downside to that choice for us. The behaviour in question might be one we are not really all that eager to change. The way the persuader can get us to comply with their request is to keep reminding us of specific consequences of non-compliance. In situations where behaviour change is designed to alleviate risk, we must believe that the risk to us is real and present. This was the approach used by the UK government in encouraging people across the country to comply with its stringent behaviour restrictions during the initial lockdown in the spring of 2020.

The government asked many people to stop seeing members of their families, to avoid going to work, to close down their businesses, hence putting their livelihoods under threat, to accept a world in which all cultural, leisure and entertainment activities were indefinitely suspended, and to keep their physical distance from other people when they did venture out. To command compliance to this degree and on such a wide scale and with little advance notice, it was necessary to go beyond mere reason and to use fear. This response in many people simultaneously was achieved by broadcasting regular messages underlining the extent of risk from the new coronavirus. Despite the statistical probability of dying from this new virus once infected, most attention was given to death rates. In reality, as a proportion of the general population, the probability of dying for most people was remote, the constant emphasis on deaths that had occurred cultivated an entirely different worldview.

Using a phenomenon variously referred to as the "availability heuristic" or "construct accessibility", frequent mentions of deaths led people to believe they were more commonly occurring than they really were. This deception might be seen by some as unethical, but in a national crisis it was a necessary evil to achieve a greater good, namely slowing the spread of this new virus, for which at the time no known and effective pharmacological interventions were available.

It is known from research with heuristics that these simple descriptive ideas about society can motivate people to change their behaviour in ways they would not have countenanced if they had considered the facts in a more reflective or systematic way. By persuading people that through changing their behaviour in specific ways and in accepting the extreme restrictions deployed by government, they would increase their personal safety.

As a further aspect of the motivation to comply, by emphasising even greater risks to specific sub-groups, such as the elderly, people would be driven to comply to safeguard others such as relatives and friends who were perceived to belong to the most "at-risk" groups. Going still further, the message asked people to comply not just for these essentially selfish but also for a greater civic good by "protecting the health services" that would be put under considerable strain by people seeking hospital treatment for this virus.

Nudging and the Pandemic

As explained above, nudging techniques might use messages or signals that encourage people to make fast assessments of situations and then to decide upon action to take often on the basis of incomplete information. Instead, decisions are guided by presumptions about the "type" of situation with which the individual is faced and to presume that specific outcomes in this case are likely to resemble outcomes believed typically to occur in such settings. This type of nudge has been labelled as System 1. In addition, there is a slower form of decision making that is encouraged (or "nudged") based on a slower and more considered form of analysis of the specific situation and its characteristics. This System 2 approach requires more cognitive effort on the part of the individual than does System 1 (De Neys, 2006; Evans & Stanovich, 2013). System 1 tends to involve more intuitive thinking and System 2 involves more analytical thinking. Both approaches can produce accurate and productive decisions and outcomes for individual (Van Gestel et al., 2020).

Although System 1 processing might seem likely to deliver less effective judgements about a risk setting than System 2 judgements, this is not invariably the case. Under conditions in which rapid-fire decisions are needed, the first system may prove to be the more effective of the two. More reflective approaches take time and when time is not available, any decisions they deliver may become available too late to be useful (Evans & Curtis-Holmes, 2005). Moreover, some writers in this field have argued that many people naturally turn to System 1 processes because they are "cognitive misers" and cannot usually motivate themselves to adopt more effortful, reflective processes (Fiske & Taylor, 2013).

On the other side of the decision-making coin, however, reliance on System 1 processing can result in biased outcomes because stereotypes can influence decisions more than situation-specific analysis (Evans et al., 2010). In the context of the coronavirus pandemic, the public needed to know how to behave to protect themselves in a situation fraught with uncertainty because the disease that was spreading rapidly was new. Hence, their political leaders had to take decisions on the back of limited knowledge. Even medical and scientific experts were on a fast-learning curve during the early stages of the pandemic.

Nudges were therefore based on limited knowledge grounded in probabilities of outcomes that could run far short of certainties. Initially, concern about surface transmission of SARS-CoV-2 led to advisories from governments about keeping physical surfaces that were likely to be touched by lots of people as clean as possible and for people themselves to wash their hands thoroughly after they had been out and in contact with lots of objects and surfaces. When it became clearer that the primary mode of transmission was airborne, the advice changed to keeping a minimum physical distance from other people unless you already lived with them.

Physical distancing signs gradually appeared in those physical spaces that remained open to people, together with handwashing signs next to supplies of hand sanitiser and eventually face-mask wearing signals. These devices offered direct, on-the-spot cues to behaviour change. More generally, however, people in general were persuaded to shift their behaviours through reflective and analytical judgements about personal risk. Risk assessments were triggered by high-profile and repeated televised government briefings and follow-on and often detailed news discussions and reports about these briefings in which progressively climbing infection, hospitali-sation and, most of all, death rates were emphasised.

Ultimately, the efficacy of nudge approaches within the context of the coronavirus pandemic must depend upon empirical proof. Theoretically, nudges have proven to be effective across a range of other behaviour change scenarios. However, the lessons learned from these earlier appli-cations turn out to be transferable to behaviour control strategy in an unprecedented global crisis cannot be presumed. Chapter 6 will revisit the application and testing of nudge theory in relation to physical distancing behaviour. Chapters 10 and 11 will then present evidence about how well this model worked in relation to public adoption of personal protective measures such as handwashing and use of face coverings and in relation to getting vaccinated.

References

Campbell-Arvai, V., Arvai, J., & Kalof, L. (2014). Motivating sustainable food choices: The role of nudges, value orientation, and information provision. *Environment and Behavior, 46*(4), 453–475.

Chapman, L. J. (1967). Illusory correlation in observational report. *Journal of Verbal Learning, 6*, 151–155.

Chen, S., & Chaiken, S. (1999). The heuristic-systematic model in its broader context. In S. Chaiken & Y. Trope (Eds.), *Dual-Process Theories in Social Psychology* (pp. 73–96). New York, NY: Guilford Press.

De Neys, W. D. (2006). Dual processing in reasoning: Two systems but one rea-soner. *Psychological Science, 17*(5), 428–433. https://doi.org/10.1111/j.1467-9280.2006.01723.x

Evans, J. S. B. T., & Curtis-Holmes, J. (2005). Rapid responding increases belief bias: Evidence for the dual-process theory of reasoning. *Thinking and Reasoning, 11*(4), 382–389. https://doi.org/10.1080/13546780542000005

Evans, J. S. B., Handley, S. J., Neilens, H., & Over, D. (2010). The influence of cognitive ability and instructional set on causal conditional inference. *The Quarterly Journal of Experimental Psychology, 63*(5), 892–909. https://doi.org/10.1080/17470210903111821

Evans, J. S. B. T., & Stanovich, K. E. (2013). Dual-process theories of higher cognition: Advancing the debate. *Perspectives on Psychological Science, 8*(3), 223–241. https://doi.org/10.1177/1745691612460685

Ferguson, N. M., Laydon, D., Nedjati-Gilani, G., et al. (2020, 16th March). *Impact of non-pharmaceutical interventions (NPIs) to reduce COVID-19 mortality and healthcare demand*. Imperial College London. https://doi.org/10.25561/77482. Available at: https://spiral.imperial.ac.uk:8443/bitstream/10044/1/77482/14/2020-03-16-COVID19-Report-9.pdf

Fiske, S. T., & Taylor, S. E. (2013). *Social Cognition: From Brains to Culture*. London, UK: SAGE.

Gunter, B. (1987). *Television and the Fear of Crime*. London, UK: John Libbey.

Haigh, M. S., & List, J. A. (2005). Do professional traders exhibit myopic loss aversion? An experimental analysis. *Journal of Finance*, 60(1), 523–534.

Kahneman, D. (2003). A perspective on judgment and choice: Mapping bounded rationality. *American Psychologist*, 58, 697–720.

Kroese, F., Marchiori, D., & de Ridder, D. (2016). Nudging healthy food choices: A field experiment at the train station. *Journal of Public Health*, 38(2), e133–e137.

Parkinson, J. A., Eccles, K. E., & Goodman, A. (2014). Positive impact by design: The Wales Centre for behaviour change. *Journal of Positive Psychology*, 9(6), 517–522.

Read, J. D. (1995). The availability heuristic in person identification: The sometimes misleading consequences of enhanced contextual information. *Applied Cognitive Psychology*, 9(2), 91–121.

Riddle, K. (2010). Always on my mind: Exploring how frequent, recent and vivid television portrayals are used in the formation of social reality judgments. *Media Psychology*, 13(2), 155–179.

Rigby, S. (2020, 12th August). COVID-19: Psychological 'nudges' change intention but not behaviour. *Science Focus*.

Saghai, Y. (2013). Salvaging the concept of nudge. *Journal of Medical Ethics*, 39(8), 487–493.

Segev, S., Fernandez, J., & Wang, W. (2015). The effects of gain versus loss message framing and point of reference on consumer responses to green advertising. *Journal of Current Issues and Research in Advertising*, 36(12), 35–51.

Sjöberg, L., & Engelberg, E. (2010). Risk perception and movies: A study of availability as a factor in risk perception. *Risk Analysis*, 30(1), 95–106.

Thaler, R., & Sunstein, C. (2009). *Nudge: Improving Decisions about Health, Wealth and Happiness*. Oxford, UK: Blackwell.

Tversky, A., & Kahneman, D. (1973). Availability: A heuristic for judging frequency and probability. *Cognitive Psychology*, 5(2), 207–232.

Tversky, A., & Kahneman, D. (1979). Prospect theory: An analysis of decision under risk. *Econometrica*, 47(2), 263–291.

Van Gestel, L. C., Adriaanse, M. A., & de Ridder, D. T. D. (2020). Do nudges make use of automatic processing? Unraveling the effects of a default nudge under type 1 and type 2 processing. *Comprehensive Results in Social Psychology*. https://doi.org/10.1080/23743603.2020.1808456

Chapter 3

Social Identity Theory and the Pandemic

In the absence of tried-and-tested, and approved, pharmaceutical measures, such as vaccines and drug therapies, governments around the world were dependent upon non-pharmaceutical interventions (NPIs) in the early stages of the COVID-19 pandemic to bring the spread of infections under control (Bonell et al., 2020; Flaxman et al., 2020). These methods did not represent a new methodology for pandemic control, but the different and extensive ways in which they were manifested around the world was a new experience for most people. These measures predominantly took the form of behaviour change. Publics in different countries were encouraged to take greater care over personal hygiene by washing their hands regularly and thoroughly, to keep surfaces clean in places visited by lots of people, to practice safer coughing and sneezing techniques, to wear face coverings, and to avoid physical spaces in which they might come into prolonged and close proximity to others. They were also advised to monitor themselves and others close to them for tell-tale symptoms and to shut themselves away if they displayed these symptoms (Drury et al., 2020).

These requests by governments, which sometimes turned into requirements underpinned by new legislation, meant suspension of large parts of people's normal lives. This had serious economic impacts on many people. It has significant psychological effects on many more. It was critical, however, that people adhered to these restrictions for their own safety and others'. There were particular tensions created in families when younger members cared for older members who did not live with them. Prohibitions on people from different households mixing socially meant that cared-for individuals were left isolated. Community action groups sprung up in some locations in which altruistic individuals proactively engaged with taking permitted actions to help those in need and isolated by these new restrictions.

More generally, it was important that, no matter how hard it was, people had to try to comply with these restrictions. Earlier theoretical models identified the potential significance of environmental signals or "nudges" and the importance internal rationalising processes within individuals in

DOI: 10.4324/9781003274308-3

controlling public behaviour. Another psychological perspective that was investigated and tested as a model for understanding better how to control public behaviour focused on group processes. The relevance of understanding such processes was illustrated in part by the community action groups already noted. More generally, however, these processes were significant in relation to the way people behave under conditions when normal community-wide rules of social engagement have been compulsorily suspended.

One important psychological construct in this context is "social identity". This concept refers to a sense of group belongingness people develop in relation to the various groups and communities of people with whom they have co-existed or pursued specific activities of mutual interest and importance. In the theory of planned behaviour which will be covered in Chapter 4, it will be seen that the perceptions people have of the responses of other people in specific behaviour change scenarios can influence whether an individual will change their own behaviour.

The group processes approach takes this idea further and examines the impact of collective group processes. The relevance of this approach can be understood when recognising that most people belong to or identify with more than one membership or reference group. The need to conform to the behavioural norms of these groups is an important driver of individuals own behavioural decisions. The willingness to conform to the action preferences of a group to which the individual belongs could overrule the behaviour changes recommendations or requirements of experts or higher authorities. Whether this does occur will depend also on the extent to which specific groups are perceived to be credible and trusted sources of influence. This point applies to groups with which individuals engage indirectly such as remote expert sources, politicians and the media, as well as to groups with which individual interacts more directly such as friends and family and work colleagues, perhaps as well as others such as special interest groups, religious institutions, and others.

Social Identity and Group Processes: Potential Relevance to Pandemic Control

People's behaviours are extensively controlled by social norms. Individuals observe the behaviour of others and might also receive advice or instruction about how to behave in different settings from members of important social groups to which they belong. These groups will include their families, neighbours, school friends and teachers, work colleagues, and co-members of sports teams and interest or social clubs or groups to which they belong. These social influences will teach individuals, from an early age, about how they are expected to behave in different situations (Smith, 2020).

Social norms can evolve organically in social groups through the interactions that take place between members over time and as they discover which behavioural practices work best for the group (Sherif, 1936). These norms then become frames of reference for individuals that they might take with them beyond the context of the group within which they first arose. Groups use their own norms to determine courses of action when dealing with new sets of circumstances (Moscovici, 1988).

During the pandemic therefore if members of their social group become infected individuals are able to learn about the new disease through their experience of it. In the context of adoption of protective devices or treatments, they might again look to the responses of other group members to help them make up their minds about whether these interventions are effective and safe (Allcott et al., 2020; Crimston & Silvanathan, 2020; Gollwitzer et al., 2020). Group reference points will also be important in helping individuals to decide whether specific authorities or expert information sources are trustworthy (Maher et al., 2020). With a behaviour such as wearing face masks, individuals may be more likely to comply when they see members of an important reference group being compliant and will be less likely to do so if this protective behaviour has been largely rejected by other group members (Neville et al., 2021).

The influence of group processes can be good or bad. This depends upon the nature of the behaviour that emerges from a group consensus about how to behave. In the middle of the 20th century, before and during the Second World War, much of the attention given to group processes focused on extremism such as the rise of the Communism and Nazism that gave rise to persecution of other groups. These examples demonstrated how, under strong and extreme group influences, individuals could be conditioned to behave in inhumane ways (Milgram, 1963). In the context of the pandemic, public behaviour showed how collectively people could come together to engage in many pro-social activities to help others in need during a time of crisis, but could also, under some group influences, adopt more selfish responses to the drive to get vaccinated (Neville & Reicher, 2020).

Important aspects of group processes theory have been the concepts of social identity and self-categorisation (Reicher et al., 2010; Spears, 2021). Individuals absorb an identity from a group that becomes integrated into their understanding of their own self (Tajfel & Turner, 1979). People can take different "identities" from different groups (e.g., their family and their work colleagues) and these will become overtly manifest through different behaviour patterns in different settings. That is, people behave differently around their families from how they behave around people they work with. Each group to which an individual belongs will have its own norms and these "rules" or "conventions" of behaviour might each influence how an individual will respond in specific social conditions. Hence compliance with behaviour change programmes will often depend upon whether surrounding group members, whose norms are the most relevant to the situation in which behaviour change is required, will have some influence over how the individual will eventually behave. For teenagers, perhaps even though mask wearing is endorsed by their parents, if it is frowned upon by the more important reference group of their peers or friends, they will probably choose not to wear a mask (Capraro & Barcelo, 2020; Levita, 2020).

With "norms", a distinction has been made between "injunctive norms" and "descriptive norms". With injunctive norms, these tend to be wrapped up in beliefs about the behaviours that have typically attracted rewards or penalties in the past (Cialdini et al., 1990, 1991). Descriptive norms derive from observations of behaviour patterns that have typically been displayed in the past and which might therefore be expected in the future. The latter experience might also have taught which behaviour patterns have proven to be the most effective (Eriksson et al., 2015).

Injunctive norms might trigger persuasive campaigns that create messages containing advice about what should or should not be done. Their effectiveness however can depend upon the behaviour of the sources of these messages. Sources must be regarded as credible and part of this reputation is based upon a perceived consistency between how the source behaves and the behaviour expected by the source of those at whom he/she has directed their message. If sources break their own rules therefore this can undermine their authority and credibility and weakens the power of their behaviour change messages (Cialdini, 2003). In fact, such inconsistency can result in those being influenced pushing back and behaving in precisely the way they were being told not to (Smith et al., 2018). Hence, when people are told to physically distance themselves from others during the pandemic by a politician who then promptly flouts his or her own advice, the public might simply ignore what they are being told to do (Steffens, 2020).

The norms that arise from membership of groups are not fixed psychological constructs. Rather, they have fluidity and can change as intra-group and inter-group exchanges cause them to adapt and evolve over time (Thomas et al., 2019). At any one time, however, a group will adhere to a specific set of beliefs and any departure from these among individual group members will be challenged. In other words, if a person joins a group there will be an expectation that they will exhibit beliefs consistent with group norms. In this way, a group will establish its own distinctive identity and will be able to distinguish itself from other groups (Reicher & Stott, 2020; Stott et al., 2012).

One other observation is that individuals will sometimes exaggerate their own compliance with specific behavioural norms. Where such behaviours are approved by a reference group, individuals will claim greater than average compliance. Where specific behaviours are disapproved, individuals will claim greater than average avoidance. This trend was found in relation to claims of compliance with pandemic-related restrictions (Fancourt et al., 2020b).

In establishing new norms, clear messages of encouragement to adopt them are important. These messages must secure social norm level changes to achieve longer-term success. Even the appearance that a few people are changing their behaviour can begin to turn others (Mortensen et al., 2019; Sparkman & Walton, 2017).

Heightening the Public's Risk Concerns

Early government messaging about the pandemic in many countries reported regularly on the case rates, hospitalisation figures and numbers of deaths from or with COVID-19. This messaging emphasised worst-case scenarios and generated a climate of threat based on an idea that everyone was at risk from this new disease. The statistical reality was that most people would not experience any symptoms or only mild ones. Few would actually die from this virus, once infected, although for older people, especially those aged over 80 and for others that had chronic health conditions, the death risk was higher. Playing on people's risk perceptions may have delivered results in terms of compliance with behavioural restrictions, but considered on its own failed, according to some psychologists, to give a complete picture of how ordinary people assessed their own circumstances during the pandemic.

When people are confronted with crisis situations that pose a direct or indirect risk to them, they seek to find out whatever they can to find ways to cope with the threat and deal with it emotionally. This support frequently comes from the social groups to which they belong. These do not simply comprise their immediate family and more distant relatives, but also various friendship groups and other communities or organisations with which they engage in their lives. These groups can provide reassurance that informs individuals and allows them to re-assess their own risks. These groups might also encourage them directly via advice, expectation or criticism of the individual's behaviour or indirectly through their own actions, to comply (or not) with the advice or instructions of the authorities. In understanding whether people will comply with their government's interventions to control the pandemic, it was essential to examine these group processes and the role they played in shaping people's responses (Cruwys, Stevens & Greenaway, 2020).

Research conducted during the pandemic showed that some government NPIs had been effective in slowing the spread of the novel coronavirus (Anderson et al., 2020; Wilder-Smith & Freedman, 2020). It was probably never going to be the case that all public behaviour would change in ways their governments might have liked during the pandemic. In some cases, people might have found it difficult, if not impossible, to abandon elderly relatives in need of their regular support because of "stay at home" rules. The personal hygiene advice hit home with many people, but not everyone diligently covered their noses when sneezing or washed their hands while singing "Happy Birthday" twice.

With an airborne disease such as COVID-19, individuals could catch the virus from anyone with whom they interacted long enough in close proximity. Hence, they might readily be infected by strangers on public transport or in a restaurant or by members of their own family with whom they share a home, if they have been mingling a lot with others (Keeling, 2005). Before the SARS-CoV-2 pandemic, analysis of previous pandemics showed that NPIs had been used and some, such as quarantining or isolating those known to be infected, were standard procedures. It would seem to make common sense that if a virus is transmitted mostly through the air from person-to-person, then limiting these interpersonal contacts across a population ought to work to slow the spread of the disease. Yet, it is not always clear precisely how much risk is presented by different physical spaces in which people physically engage with each other and so it is not always clear just how effective closure of these spaces might be (Mao & Yang, 2012).

Social network analysis, a procedure that can be subsumed under a "group processes" perspective tries to measure the volume of contacts individuals have with others in different spaces. This can be used to track changes in the volume of potential human-to-human interactions. Individuals that interact with large networks of others in tightly clustered spaces can experience a rapid spread of an airborne disease and contribute to societal transmission levels more than would individuals with smaller contact networks. There is further evidence that in tightly clustered networks, transmission rates can fall away as quickly they initially evolved (Keeling, 2005). The same may not be as true of individuals with smaller networks with far less membership clustering.

In nudge approaches, the behaviour of individuals can be influenced through often subtle environmental signals that might comprise physical signs in different settings (e.g., floor markings designed to keep people two metres apart) or messaging that frequently contains cues relating to risk. Trying directly to encourage people to respond to risk assessment by changing their behaviour might be significantly enhanced, if risks and risk assessments are considered within broader social contexts. Success in persuading people to change their behaviour will depend in part on the way they normally behave in different settings.

These pre-existing behaviour patterns will, in turn, be influenced by the social groups with which individuals engage or in which they have an identifiable membership. Social norms of conduct, prescribed by membership groups, that are also reference sources when individuals seek to decide on the appropriate ways to behave, are influential in this context. Individuals do not just obtain rules about behaviour through these group dynamics, but also find that group interactions define their own social identities (Tajfel & Turner, 1979; Turner et al., 1987). Social identities have been invoked as important psychological factors that underpin people's health risk behaviours (Cruwys, Greenaway et al., 2020).

Concerns about Public Compliance Commitment

There were doubts among some governments and experts that national populations would be willing to accept far-reaching restrictions on their behaviours (Reicher et al., 2020). Research conducted on other national and international disasters and emergencies had shown that people could show great resilience and that they would find new ways of dealing with circumstances in which normal, everyday behaviours were not possible. People would also often work together in collectives or groups from which would arise spontaneous mutual help programmes (Drury et al., 2019).

In setting out a perspective for understanding, further inquiry into and learning about the pandemic, the group processes approach makes reference to people's membership of different groups or social categories and what these memberships might mean in terms of the social values, beliefs and attitudes an individual might hold and the choice they might make in respect of behaviour change.

A pandemic usually represents a time of crisis. The 2020–2021 SARS-CoV-2 pandemic was unprecedented for most people and nations in terms of the scale and severity of its effects. While lessons could be learned from how people had responded during other major catastrophes such as earthquakes, floods, hurricanes and volcanic eruptions, epidemics and pandemics could take place over longer time frames. The COVID-19 pandemic had the added characteristic of being felt all around the world and represented a crisis in which potentially everyone could become a victim. During this crisis, virtually all members of nations affected had to change their usual behaviour patterns. Getting them to do this willingly meant instilling in them a sense of threat and of social responsibility. Threat could motivate behaviour change motivated by the need for self-protection and civic or social responsibility meant being concerned about the welfare of others.

When people feel under threat, their behaviour can change dramatically and quickly and not always rationally. In settings of this kind, some people will enter a panic state (Clarke, 2002). This behaviour is underpinned by fear, but in some fear-evoking situations, a fear response is entirely proportional to the risk or danger being perceived. In other settings, the fear can drive a disproportionate response as the fear that is triggered goes beyond what is optimal to trigger appropriate behaviour. The practical problem confronted by anyone researching this phenomenon is knowing when fear is excessive rather than appropriate (Sime, 1980).

During the COVID-19 pandemic, stories emerged that people in the United Kingdom were "panic-buying" regular household products. There were several possible reasons underpinning this behaviour. Some people were concerned that if new restrictions meant they would have to remain at home for long periods, they needed to stockpile goods. Another reason was that people thought supply chains would be disrupted and that there would be shortages of some products. Another factor might have been that they observed others doing this, so they felt they needed to do likewise. In the last case, their behaviour was driven by individuals' perceptions of others which possibly generated a mindset that they needed to conform by doing the same.

In times of crisis, members of the public can become more acutely attuned to risks and threats. Even when these outcomes are statistically rare, they nevertheless exhibit heightened sensitivity to specific signs of crises and the effects they could have. Public overreaction during times of emergencies is not unknown and in itself it can represent a significant safety risk to those involved (Forsyth, 1983). As we saw earlier in this book, this phenomenon has been explained in terms of the "availability heuristic". Rare events seem less rare if they attain a high enough profile even for a short duration. Yet, individuals can also underestimate specific personal risks by believing that other people are at greater risk than themselves. They become overly optimistic about their own security (Atwood & Major, 2000; Kinsey et al., 2019).

The right perspective in dealing with or responding to a crisis can be promoted by prior experience. Learning lessons from history can inform individuals and authorities in terms of how to behave in the face of a new emergency situation. While some threats might seem remote and rare, regular reminders that they might not be can change dramatically and fundamentally the way they are perceived by people (Becker et al., 2017; Wormwood et al., 2016).

Another aspect to risk and threat perceptions that can, in turn, shape public behaviour, is a social identity reaction whereby the identity that an individual ascribes to themselves on the basis of a specific group membership might also sensitise them to how different they are from others. If specific risks have been linked in public minds to a specific group, such as terrorism in the West with Muslims, all members of the outgroup (Muslims) could be seen as potentially risky and this will influence how other respond to them (Staple et al., 1994).

These social category perceptions can also determine whether a specific threat is relevant to an individual. In the context of COVID-19, the virus was found early on to be a higher risk to older people than to younger people. That is, older people were more likely to display symptoms, they were more likely to be hospitalised or to need intensive care treatment once infected, and had a higher risk of dying from the disease. These risks were very low to miniscule for very young people for whom behavioural restrictions could therefore have been regarded as less relevant. If they are very unlikely to get ill from this virus, why should they curtail their normal, everyday behaviours? Put simply, the behavioural restrictions, such as social isolation had relevance to older people, but not to younger people (Cruwys, Stevens & Greenaway, 2020).

These reactions could have important repercussions on the extent to which people adhere to behavioural restrictions imposed upon them by their government. If new behaviour regulations are perceived to be of questionable relevance, the public will need further persuasion to comply. Telling people to stay at home, for example, might be a difficult message for some to swallow not just because for some, it might pose caring or financial difficulties for them. Under the theory of planned behaviour, "which is examined in the next chapter" people must believe they can change their behaviour "perceived behavioural control", If people believe they cannot change their behaviour, behavioural compliance will be less likely. Under the group processes perspective, the lack of perceived group relevance will cause people's willingness to adopt new behaviour patterns to be weakened (Foster, 2020).

Within the social identity and group processes perspectives, perceptions of sources are important factors. It is critical that any sources behind messages to people to change their behaviours are regarded by message recipients as credible and trustworthy. The messages being communicated must also make sense and offer information that is regarded as relevant and consistent. In the United Kingdom, at the outset of the pandemic, trust in the government was high (Fancourt et al., 2020a). This state of affairs undoubtedly played an important part in engineering widespread public compliance with the extensive behavioural restrictions of the first national lockdown. Once again, the trust in a message source will often be determined by whether recipients perceive the source as a co-member of a shared group. The more, message recipients identify with the message source, because both are seen to share a common social identity, the more a behaviour change will be accepted (Haslam, 2020; Turner, 1991).

Self-Determination, Self-Identity and Behaviour Change

Psychologists have found that public compliance with behaviour messages or change campaigns is most likely to be internalised and accepted by people when it is communicated with clarity and in a caring manner. When governments issue guidelines concerning how people must ideally behave given a specific set of circumstances, such as a pandemic, those on the receiving end of such messages must feel that they have some control still over how they behave. New behavioural rules must present a framework for public behaviour that has people's best interests at its core. The public must readily perceive this framework as inviting a partnership between themselves and those in authority. Furthermore, if the behaviour changes present challenges to people, authorities must indicate how they will help and support these changes (Martela et al., 2021).

According to the perspective of Self-Determination Theory, people must retain a sense that they can still determine their own behaviour to some degree albeit within a tighter set of parameters than they had been used to previously. If this balance can be struck effectively, then public compliance is more likely to follow.

In effect, the objective is to achieve voluntary compliance among the public. In the context of a pandemic, people do not need to be frightened out of their wits. While some degree of fear might help to motivate behaviour, it is more important to ensure that people understand why the government has taken specific steps to control or restrict normal public behaviour. The rules therefore need to be clear and perceived as relevant and reasonable given prevailing circumstances (Aelterman et al., 2019). People need to know what they just do and what they should avoid doing, but also need to believe they still have some autonomy over choices about compliance (Ntoumanis et al., 2021; Slemp et al., 2018). Excessive centralised control over public behaviour with little latitude given to people to decide on how they behave can lead to defiance or reactance whereby new rules and regulations are rejected (Van Petegem et al., 2015; Weinstein et al., 2020).

Self-determination can work alongside social identity. Social identity is often influenced in significant ways by group processes. Individuals join groups that become reference points for how to behave. Social determination theory has been used to understand how people behave during times of natural disasters such as earthquakes and tsunamis and then in turn how appropriate behavioural responses to these incidents can be cultivated (Drury, 2018; Drury et al., 2019).

In the context of the coronavirus pandemic, people engaged in various protective behaviours such as handwashing and physical distancing but may have done so for varying reasons. Some people internalised the advice relating to why these behaviours were good practice to control personal risk of infection. For others, compliance with these behaviours occurred because others around pressurised them. It is important to distinguish therefore between people who behaved a certain way because they wanted to from those that did so because they were made to.

The nature of the motivation underpinning the adoption of protective behaviour is important in terms of whether compliance will occur and will persist over time. For those that have internalised motives that drive protective behaviour, compliance is likely to persist even in the absence of external policing. Where individuals need constant reminders to take protective steps, external monitoring is needed together with periodic coercion (Morbee et al., 2021). Individuals also need to feel that they have made their choices freely and that they are able to change their behaviours in ways that will prove to be effective (Cantarero et al., 2021; van der Kaap-deeder et al., 2021).

Social Identity and Health Risk

When people are asked to define who they are, they will use descriptions of how they perceive themselves as individuals and they will also frequently make reference to the social groups of which they are members (Turner et al., 1987). Group membership has been confirmed by research the world over as a central aspect of self-identity definition (Haslam, 2014). People make reference to the people with whom they engage in organised processes and on more informal occasions in forming their views about the world and more specifically in the context of this book in terms of their judgements about personal risks. When deciding on the significance of potential risks, comparisons will often be made between a position concerning a group to which the individual belongs (an *ingroup*) and groups to which the individual does not belong (*outgroups*).

Ingroups will command greater trust than outgroups. This will be especially true when risk assessments are being made. A response to a potential threat that is endorsed or made by an ingroup will tend to be seen as less risky than one made by an outgroup. Groups to which an individual belongs or with which they identify or aspire to belong will exert stronger influence over an individual's behaviour than groups that hold no interest for them. Individuals will conform to ingroup norms but not to outgroup norms (Neighbors et al., 2010; Stevens et al., 2019). In the context of COVID-19, therefore, compliance with government-imposed behaviour restrictions will usually be strengthened when an ingroup exhibits compliance and invites its members to do so. Likewise, if an ingroup decided to lobby against pandemic-related rules, this action would provoke increased likelihood that individuals that belong to that group will follow suit. The same action made by an outgroup would not influence in the same way any individual lacking identification with or membership of that group (Ferris et al., 2019).

Group Membership Effects

People's risk-taking can be determined by a multitude of factors. Research has shown that people with different personality types may be more or less prone to take risks. There is also evidence that the social groups to which people belong are also relevant in this context. People will weigh up risks on the basis of relevant information they receive about outcome probabilities of events. The extent to which the information they receive is believed or perceived to be credible will often depend upon its source. Sources may then be judged in terms of whether they are part of an ingroup or outgroup. Ingroup sources will generally be treated as more credible than outgroup sources and this means they will usually be more influential.

When it comes to taking actions to mitigate against risks, ingroup sources will be important influences. Indeed, behaviours performed by their other ingroup members are more likely to be adopted individuals as compared to when those same behaviours are performed only by outgroup members (Greenaway & Cruwys, 2019; Zhai & Du, 2020).

There are potential downsides to ingroup influences. If their reference ingroup makes bad choices, individuals might still engage in those high-risk options themselves. In a health context, this response could be critical if it places the individual at even greater risk of harm. Yet, this situation can be difficult to counter through public policy. When people at a mass gathering hear speeches encouraging them to behave in a certain way, they will be more likely to comply when they perceive those around as fellow ingroups members than as strangers who are members of an outgroup (Hult Khazaie & Khan, 2019).

One interesting illustration of this phenomenon occurred in a study that found that people's perceptions of the potential health harms of alcohol consumption regarded drinking beer as less dangerous when presented with beer in cans garnished with the colours of their own university as opposed to a rival university (Loersch & Bartholow, 2011). Elsewhere, officers from the armed forces and police force were more likely to jump into freezing water when accompanied by others with whom they shared a work-related identity (Firing & Laberg, 2012).

Studies of the effects of group membership on health-related behaviour have shown that the health risks that individuals will take can be influenced directly by group processes. Participants in one experiment said that they felt the health risk posed by tissues used by someone with a cold was greater when that person was identified as an ingroup member than when they were shown to be an outgroup member. Other studies found that individuals were prepared to stay longer at an art festival in which dismembered animal carcasses with close by when fellow attendees were ingroup as opposed to outgroup members. On another occasion, individuals showed they were more willing to shake hands with a person who had a rash on their hands when they learned he was a member of their political party as compared to having membership of a different party (Cruwys et al., 2020).

Trust in Sources and Group Processes Effects

People's responses to public health policies designed to slow the spread of a pandemic will depend upon the judgements they make about the information they have received about how they should behave and about where that information comes from. This means that, at a fundamental level, the public must believe and therefore trust information sources. What people learn about a new disease will be informed by factual information delivered by experts and also by stories about people made ill by it and whether they recovered. People can also learn from their social networks and their beliefs can be powerfully influenced by social groups they belong to or aspire to join.

People can display strong emotional reactions to a threat such as a new disease in addition to their cognitive appraisal of risks (van Leeuwen & Petersen, 2018). Once again, group membership can play a part in controlling this type of emotional reaction. While a health issue might give rise to unpleasant visceral responses, these responses might be less severe when reported for ingroup members as opposed to outgroup members. One example is that the smell of a soiled baby is perceived as less acute with a person's own child as compared to other people's children (Case et al., 2006). Ingroup members are generally regarded as posing a less serious risk by other members than did outgroup members when both suffer from the same health problem (Faulkner et al., 2004; Steffens et al., 2019).

A sweaty T-shirt is an object many people would be unwilling to touch unless perhaps they had been the ones wearing it. Research showed, however, that students were less disgusted by such a T-shirt when it bore the emblem of their university as compared to a rival university or when it was made known that the shirt belonged to a member of their own university as compared to a member of a different university. Then, if they had been made to touch the T-shirt, they walked more swiftly over to a bottle of hand sanitiser to clean their hands when the shirt was identified as belonging to their own university rather than a rival university (Reicher et al., 2016). This type of research serves to illustrate how people's judgements about risks and emotional responses to unpleasant experiences can be moderated when they learn that members of an ingroup were more involved than members of an outgroup.

Some psychologists have therefore argued that these experiments and their findings hold important lessons for public policy makers that are involved in creating plans for changing people's behaviour patterns during a time of national crisis. One of the ways in which this psychological science evidence might be important is in relation to modelling how people might behave in specific behaviour-restrictive circumstances. When individuals turn to ingroups for guidance on how to behave and, in particular, for signals about how ingroups have already reacted to restrictions themselves, it is important to know how these groups collectively have behaved. Ingroups will exert more influence over individuals than strangers. This means that even suggestions about how people in general have responded to government advice could hold little currency, as a source of influence for some people who turn first to a specific reference group for the lead on how they should behave themselves.

It is important to persuade the public that adherence to specified behavioural restrictions is essential not only to protect themselves but also to protect others. Following the lessons learned from research on group processes and social identity, these "others" would be best portrayed in terms of being "close contacts" rather than diffuse and ill-defined "others". Appeals to collective responsibility are likely to work best when the "collective" is described as "close or vulnerable family members" or "loved ones" (Everett et al., 2020; Jordan et al., 2020).

The alternative to voluntary action on the part of the public, perhaps motivated by a sense of collective civic responsibility or simply by individuals' perceptions of personal risk or threat, would be coercive methods of behavioural compliance. These do not invariably work well, however. They can generate psychological reactance and be rejected by those being subjugated. When people recognise a need to take personal steps to safeguard themselves and others and see other people doing the same, a sense of shared group responsibility can emerge that has a powerful effect on the way people then behave (Carter et al., 2013a). This shared behavioural responsibility can relieve public anxiety about threatening circumstances and motivate continued public adherence to any ongoing restrictions (Carter et al., 2013b, 2014).

In the United Kingdom, adherence to physical distancing restrictions and the instruction to stay at home as much as possible was high. Adherence to other associated rules such as socially isolating when symptomatic or having been in contact with someone who was, tended to be lower (Smith et al., 2020). As will become clear from the discussion in the next chapter, proponents of the "theory of planned behaviour" would have argued here that non-compliers could have been unable to contemplate isolating if that meant staying off work which they were financially not able to afford. This position was recognised within the group processes framework. Non-compliance might also have occurred because people did not always understand the precise rules around social isolation (Webster et al., 2020). The high levels of compliance observed in the United Kingdom across the first national lockdown and then later when further restrictions were introduced indicated that the public were willing to suspend their normal lives in the service of a greater good. The idea that everyone was in this together and that most others were being compliant, and especially those with whom individuals personally identified was one factor of influence in play, but probably an important one (Drury et al., 2020).

References

Aelterman, N., Vansteenkiste, M., Haerens, L., Soenens, B., Fontaine, J. R., & Reeve, J. (2019). Toward an integrative and fine-grained insight in motivating and demotivating teaching styles: The merits of a circumplex approach. *Journal of Educational Psychology*, 111(3), 497–521. https://doi.org/10.1037/edu0000293

Allcott, H., Boxell, L., Conway, J. C., Gentzkow, M., Thaler, M., & Yang, D. Y. (2020). Polarization and public health: Partisan differences in social distancing during the coronavirus pandemic. *Journal of Public Economics*, *191*, 104254. https://doi.org/10.2139/ssrn.3570274

Anderson, R. M., Heesterbeek, H., Klinkenberg, D., & Hollingsworth, T. D. (2020). How will country-based mitigation measures influence the course of the COVID-19 epidemic? *The Lancet*, *395*, 931–934. https://doi.org/10.1016/S0140-6736(20)30567-5

Atwood, L. E., & Major, A. M. (2000). Optimism, pessimism, and communication behavior in response to an earthquake prediction. *Public Understanding of Science*, *9*(4), 417–432.

Becker, J. S., Paton, D., Johnston, D. M., Ronan, K. R., & McClure, J. (2017). The role of prior experience in informing and motivating earthquake preparedness. *International Journal of Disaster Risk Reduction*, *22*, 179–193.

Bonell, C., Michie, S., Reicher, S., West, R., Bear, L., Yardley, L., et al. (2020). Harnessing behavioural science in public health campaigns to maintain 'social distancing' in response to the COVID-19 pandemic: Key principles. *Journal of Epidemiology and Community Health*, *74*(8), 617–619.

Cantarero, K., Wijnand, A., van Tilburg, P. , & Smoktunowitz, E. (2021). Affirming basic psychological needs promotes mental well-being during the COVID-19 outbreak. *Social Psychological and Personality Science*, *12*(5), 821–824.

Capraro, V., & Barcelo, H. (2020). The effect of messaging and gender on intentions to wear a face covering to slow down COVID-19 transmission. [Preprint] Retrieved from: https://psyarxiv.com/tg7vz/

Carter, H., Drury, J., Rubin, G. J., Williams, R., & Amlôt, R. (2013a). Communication during mass casualty decontamination: Highlighting the gaps. *International Journal of Emergency Service*, *2*, 29–48.

Carter, H., Drury, J., Rubin, G. J., Williams, R., & Amlôt, R. (2013b). The effect of communication on anxiety and compliance during mass decontamination. *Disaster Prevention Management*, *22*, 132–147.

Carter, H., Drury, J., Rubin, G. J., Williams, R., & Amlôt, R. (2014). Effective responder communication improves efficiency and psychological outcomes in a mass decontamination field experiment: Implications for public behaviour in the event of a chemical incident. *PLoS One*, *9*, e89846.

Case, T. I., Repacholi, B. M., & Stevenson, R. J. (2006). My baby doesn't smell as bad as yours: The plasticity of disgust. *Evolution and Human Behavior*, *27*, 357–365. https://doi.org/10.1016/j.evolhumbehav.2006.03.003

Cialdini, R. B. (2003). Crafting normative messages to protect the environment. *Current Directions in Psychological Science*, *12*(4), 105–109.

Cialdini, R. B., Kallgren, C. A., & Reno, R. R. (1991). A focus theory of normative conduct: A theoretical refinement and reevaluation of the role of norms in human behaviour. In M. P. Zanna (Ed.), *Advances in Experimental Social Psychology* (Vol. 24, pp. 201–233). Cambridge, MA: Academic Press.

Cialdini, R. B., Reno, R. R., & Kallgren, C. A. (1990). A focus theory of normative conduct: Recycling the concept of norms to reduce littering in public places. *Journal of Personality and Social Psychology*, *58*, 1015–1026. https://doi.org/1 0.1037/0022-3514.58.6.1015

Clark, C., Davila, A., Regis, M., & Kraus, S. (2020). Predictors of COVID-19 voluntary compliance behaviors: An international investigation. *Global Transition*, 2, 76–82.

Clarke, L. (2002). Panic: Myth or reality? *Contexts*, 1(3), 21–26.

Crimston, C., & Silvanathan, H. P. (2020). Polarisation. In J. Jetten, S. D. Reicher, A. A. Haslam, & T. Cruwys (Eds.), *Together Apart: The Psychology of COVID-19* (pp. 107– 112). Thousand Oaks, CA: SAGE.

Cruwys, T., Greenaway, K., Ferris, L. J., Rathbone, J., Saeri, A. K., Williams, E., Parker, S. L., Change, M. X. L., Croft, N., Bingley, W., & Grace, L. (2020). When trust goes wrong: A social identity model of risk taking. *Journal of Personality and Social Psychology*. https://doi.org/10.1037/pspi0000243

Cruwys, T., Stevens, M., & Greenaway, K. H. (2020). A social identity perspective on COVID-19: Health risk is affected by shared group membership. *British Journal of Social Psychology*, 59(3), 584–593.

Cruwys, T., Stevens, M., Platow, M. J., Drury, J., Williams, E., Kelly, A. J., & Weekes, M. (2020). Risk-taking that signals trust increases social identification. *Social Psychology*. https://doi.org/10.1027/1864-9335/a000417.

Drury, J. (2018). The role of social identity processes in mass emergency behaviour: An integrative review. *European Review of Social Psychology*, 29(1), 38–81. https://doi.org/10.1080/10463283.2018.1471948

Drury, J., Carter, H., Cocking, C., Ntontis, E., Tekin Guven, S., & Amlôt, R. (2019). Facilitating collective resilience in the public in emergencies: Twelve re-commendations based on the social identity approach. *Front Public Health*, 2019(7), 141.

Drury, J., Carter, H., Ntontis, E., & Guven, S. T. (2020). Public behaviour in response to the COVID-19 pandemic: Understanding the role of group processes. *British Journal of Psychology Open*, 7(1), e11. https://doi.org/10.1192/bjo.2020.139

Drury, J., Reicher, S., & Stott, C. (2020). From me to we: In an emergency, col-lectivise to survive. *Novara Media*. https://novaramedia.com/2020/03/22/from-me-to-we-in-an-emergency-collectivize-to-survive/

Eriksson, K., Strimling, P., & Coultas, J. C. (2015). Bidirectional associations be-tween descriptive and injunctive norms. *Organizational Behavior and Human Decision Processes*, 129, 59–69. https://doi.org/10.1016/j.obhdp.2014.09.011

Everett, J. A. C. et al. (2020). The effectiveness of moral messages on public health behavioural intentions during the COVID-19 pandemic. *PsyArXiv Preprints*.

Fancourt, D., Bu, F., Mak, H. W., & Steptoe, A. (2020a). Covid-19 social study. *Results Release 3. University College London*. https://b6bdcb03-332c-4ff9-8b9d-28f9c957493a.filesusr.com/ugd/3d9db5_13e8d6ef4dd34caf94a7a7b9ae359c95.pdf

Fancourt, D., Steptoe, A., & Wright, L. (2020b). The Cummings effect: Politics, trust, and behaviours during the COVID-19 pandemic. *Lancet*, 396, 464–465.

Faulkner, J., Schaller, M., Park, J. H., & Duncan, L. A. (2004). Evolved disease-avoidance mechanisms and contemporary xenophobic attitudes. *Group Processes & Intergroup Relations*, 7, 333–353. https://doi.org/10.1177/1368430204046142

Ferris, L. J., Radke, H. R. M., Walter, Z. C., & Crimston, C. R. (2019). Divide and conquer? Identity, threat, and moral justification of violence at the G20. *Australian Journal of Psychology*. https://doi.org/10.1111/ajpy.12249

Firing, K., & Laberg, K. C. (2012). Personal characteristics and social identity as predictors of risk taking among military officers: An empirical study. *International Journal of Management*, 29, 86–98.

Flaxman, S., Mishra, S., Gandy, A., Unwin, H. J. T., Mellan, T. A., Coupland, H., et al. (2020). Estimating the effects of non-pharmaceutical interventions on COVID-19 in Europe. *Nature*, 584, 257–261.

Forsyth, D. R. (1983). *An Introduction to Group Dynamics*. Pacific Grove, CA: Thomson Brooks/Cole Publishing.

Foster, L. (2020). Coronavirus: Young men 'More Likely to Ignore Lockdown'. *BBC News*. https://www.bbc.co.uk/news/health-52587368

Gollwitzer, A., Martel, C., Brady, W. J., Parnaments, P., Freedman, I. G., Knowles, E. D., & van Bavel, J. J. (2020). Partisan differences in physical distancing predict infections and mortality during the coronavirus pandemic. *Nature Human Behaviour*, 4, 1186–1197. https://psyarxiv.com/t3yxa/

Greenaway, K. H., & Cruwys, T. (2019). The source model of group threat: Responding to internal and external threats. *American Psychologist*, 74, 218–231. https://doi.org/10.1037/amp0000321

Haslam, S. A. (2014). Making good theory practical: Five lessons for an Applied Social Identity Approach to challenges of organizational, health, and clinical psychology. *British Journal of Social Psychology*, 53, 1–20. https://doi.org/1 0.1111/bjso.12061

Haslam, S. A. (2020). Leadership. In J. Jetten, D. D. Reicher, S. A. Haslam, & T. Cruwys (Eds.), *Together Apart: The Psychology of Covid-19*. London, UK: SAGE.

Hult Khazaie, D., & Khan, S. S. (2019). Shared social identification in mass gatherings lowers health risk perceptions via lowered disgust. *British Journal of Social Psychology*, 59(4), 839–856. https://doi.org/10.1111/bjso.12362

Jordan, J., Yoeli, E., & Rand, D. G. (2020). Don't get it or don't spread it? Comparing self-interested versus prosocially framed COVID-19 prevention messaging. https://doi.org/10.31234/osf.io/yuq7x

Keeling, M. (2005). The implications of network structure for epidemic dynamics. *Theoretical Population Biology*, 67, 1–8. https://doi.org/10.1016/j.tpb.2004. 08.002

Kinsey, M. J., Gwynne, S. M. V., Kuligowski, E. D., & Kinateder, M. (2019). Cognitive biases within decision making during fire evacuations. *Fire Technology*, 55(2), 465–485.

Levita, L. (2020). Initial research findings on the impact of COVID-19 on the well-being of young people aged 13 to 24 in the UK. *COVID-19 Psychological Research Consortium (C19PRC)*. https://drive.google.com/file/d/1AOc0wCPqv2gfFSQ_DVmw12vrqQK01z0V/view

Loersch, C., & Bartholow, B. D. (2011). The color of safety: Ingroup-associated colors make beer safer. *Journal of Experimental Social Psychology*, 47(1), 190–194. https://doi.org/10.1016/j.jesp.2010.09.001

Maher, P. J., MacCarron, P. , & Quayle, M. (2020). Mapping public health responses with attitude networks: The emergence of opinion-based groups in the UK's early COVID-19 response phase. *The British Journal of Social Psychology*, 59(3), 641–652. https://doi.org/10.1111/bjso.12396

Mao, L., & Yang, Y. (2012). Coupling infectious diseases, human preventive behavior, and networks – a conceptual framework for epidemic modeling.

Social Science and Medicine, 74, 167–175. https://doi.org/10.1016/j.socscimed.2011.10.012

Martela, F., Hankonen, N., Ryan, R. M., & Vansteenkiste, M. (2021). Motivating voluntary compliance to behavioural restrictions: Self-determination theory–based checklist of principles for COVID-19 and other emergency communications. *European Review of Social Psychology*. https://doi.org/10.1080/10463283.2020.1857082

Milgram, S. (1963). Behavioral study of obedience. *Journal of Abnormal and Social Psychology, 67*(4), 371–378. https://doi.org/10.1037/h0040525

Morbee, S., Vermots, B., Waterschoot, J. , & Dieleman, L. (2021). Adherence to COVID-19 measures: The critical role of autonomous motivation on a short- and long-term basis. *Motivation Science, 7*(4). doi: 10.1037/mot0000250

Mortensen, C. R., Neel, R., Cialdini, R. B., Jaeger, C. M., Jacobson, R. P., & Ringel, M. M. (2019). Trending norms: A lever for encouraging behaviors performed by the minority. *Social Psychological and Personality Science, 10*, 201–210. https://doi.org/10.1177/1948550617734615

Moscovici, S. (1988). Notes towards a description of social representations. *European Journal of Social Psychology, 18*(3), 211–250. https://doi.org/10.1002/ejsp.2420180303

Neighbors, C., LaBrie, J. W., Hummer, J. F., Lewis, M. A., Lee, C. M., Desai, S., … Larimer, M. E. (2010). Group identification as a moderator of the relationship between perceived social norms and alcohol consumption. *Psychology of Addictive Behaviors, 24*, 522–528. https://doi.org/10.1037/a0019944

Neville, F. G., & Reicher, S. (2020). Crowds. In J. Jetten, S. D. Reicher, A. A. Haslam, & T. Cruwys (Eds.), *Together Apart: The Psychology of COVID-19* (pp. 75–79). Thousand Oaks, CA: SAGE.

Neville, F. G., Templeton, A., Smith, J. R. , & Louis, W. R. (2021). Social norms, social identities, and the COVID-19 pandemic: Theory and recommendations. *Social and Personality Psychology Compass*.

Ntoumanis, N., Ng, J. Y., Prestwich, A., Quested, E., Hancox, J. E., Thøgersen-Ntoumani, C., Deci, E. L., Ryan, R. M., Lonsdale, C., & Williams, G. C. (2021). A meta-analysis of self-determination theory-informed intervention studies in the health domain: Effects on motivation, health behavior, physical, and psychological health. *Health Psychology Review, 15*(2), 214–244. https://doi.org/10.1080/17437199.2020.1718529

Reicher, S., Drury, J., & Stott, C. (2020). The two psychologies and coronavirus. *The Psychologist*. https://thepsychologist.bps.org.uk/two-psychologies-and-coronavirus

Reicher, S., Spears, R., & Haslam, S. A. (2010). The social identity approach in social psychology. In M. S. Wetherell & C. T. Mohanty (Eds.), *Sage Identities Handbook* (pp. 45–62). Thousand Oaks, CA: SAGE.

Reicher, S., & Stott, C. (2020). On order and disorder during the COVID-19 pandemic. *British Journal of Social Psychology, 59*(3), 694–702. https://doi.org/10.1111/bjso.12398

Reicher, S. D., Templeton, A., Neville, F., Ferrari, L., & Drury, J. (2016). Core disgust is attenuated by ingroup relations. *Proceedings of the National Academy of Sciences USA, 113*, 2631–2635. https://doi.org/10.1073/pnas.1517027113

Sherif, M. (1936). *The Psychology of Social Norms*. New York, NY: Harper and Row.

Sime, J. D. (1980). The concept of "panic". In D. Cantor (Ed.), *Fires and Human Behaviour* (pp. 63–81), Oxford, UK: Wiley.

Slemp, G. R., Kern, M. L., Patrick, K. J., & Ryan, R. M. (2018). Leader autonomy support in the workplace: A meta-analytic review. *Motivation and Emotion*, 42(5), 706–724. https://doi.org/10.1007/s11031-018-9698-y

Smith, J. R. (2020). Group norms. In O. Braddick (Ed.), *Oxford Research Encyclopaedia of Psychology*. Oxford, UK: Oxford University Press. https://doi.org/10.1093/acrefore/9780190236557.013.453

Smith, J. R., Louis, W. R., & Abraham, C. (2018). When and how does normative feedback reduce intentions to drink irresponsibly? An experimental investigation. *Addiction Research & Theory*, 26, 256–266. https://doi.org/10.1080/16066359.2017.1359572

Smith, L. E., Amlôt, R., Lambert, H., Oliver, I., Robin, C., Yardley, L., et al. (2020). Factors associated with adherence to self-isolation and lockdown measures in the UK: A cross-sectional survey. *Public Health*, 187, 21–52.

Sparkman, G., & Walton, G. M. (2017). Dynamic norms promote sustainable behavior, even if it is counternormative. *Psychological Science*, 28, 1663–1674. https://doi.org/10.1177/0956797617719950

Spears, R. (2021). Social influence and group identity. *Annual Review of Psychology*, 72, 367–390. https://doi.org/10.1146/annurev-psych-070620-111818

Staple, D. A., Reicher, S. D., & Spears, R. (1994). Social identity, availability and the perception of risk. *Social Cognition*, 12(1), 1–17.

Steffens, N. K. (2020). Compliance and followership during COVID. In J. Jetten, S. D. Reicher, A. A. Haslam, & T. Cruwys (Eds.), *Together Apart: The Psychology of COVID-19* (pp. 31–35). Thousand Oaks, CA: SAGE.

Steffens, N. K., Slade, E. L., Stevens, M., Haslam, S. A., & Rees, T. (2019). Putting the 'we' into workout: The association of identity leadership with exercise class attendance and effort, and the mediating role of group identification and comfort. *Psychology of Sport and Exercise*, 45, 101544. https://doi.org/10.1016/j.psychsport.2019.101544

Stevens, M., Rees, T., & Polman, R. (2019). Social identification, exercise participation, and positive exercise experiences: Evidence from parkrun. *Journal of Sports Sciences*, 37, 221–228. https://doi.org/10.1080/02640414.2018.1489360

Stott, C., Hoggett, J., & Pearson, G. (2012). 'Keeping the peace': Social identity, procedural justice and the policing of football crowds. *British Journal of Criminology*, 52(2), 381–399. https://doi.org/10.1093/bjc/azr076

Tajfel, H., & Turner, J. C. (1979). An integrative theory of intergroup conflict. In W. G. Austin & S. Worehel (Eds.), *The Social Psychology of Intergroup Relations* (pp. 33–47). Monterey, CA: Brooks/Cole.

Templeton, A., Guven, S. T., Hoerst, C., Vestergren, S., Davidson, L., Ballentyne, S., et al. (2020). Inequalities and identity processes in crises: Recommendations for facilitating safe response to the COVID-19 pandemic. *British Journal of Social Psychology*, 59(3), 674–685.

Thomas, E. F., McGarty, C., Stuart, A., Smith, L. G. E., & Bourgeois, L. (2019). Reaching consensus promotes the internalization of commitment to social change.

Group Processes & Intergroup Relations, 22(5), 615–630. https://doi.org/10.11 77/1368430218780320

Turner, J. C. (1991). *Social Influence*. Pacific Grove, CA: Thomson Brooks/Cole Publishing.

Turner, J. C., Hogg, M. A., Oakes, P. J., Reicher, S. D., & Wetherell, M. S. (1987). *Rediscovering the Social Group: A Self-Categorization Theory*. Oxford, UK: Blackwell.

van der Kaap-Deeder, J., Vermote, B., Waterschoot, J., Soenens, B., Morbée, S. , & Vansteenkiste, M. (2021). The role of ego integrity and despair in older adults' well-being during the COVID-19 crisis: The mediating role of need-based experiences. European Journal of Ageing, 19(1), 1-13. Advance online publication. https://doi.org/10.1007/s10433-021-00610-0

van Leeuwen, F., & Petersen, M. B. (2018). The behavioral immune system is designed to avoid infected individuals, not outgroups. *Evolution and Human Behavior, 39,* 26–34. https://doi.org/10.1016/j.evolhumbehav.2017.12.003

Van Petegem, S., Soenens, B., Vansteenkiste, M., & Beyers, W. (2015). Rebels with a cause? Adolescent defiance from the perspective of reactance theory and self-determination theory. *Child Development, 86*(3), 903–918. https://doi.org/1 0.1111/cdev.12355

Webster, R. K., Brooks, S. K., Smith, L. E., Woodland, L., Wessely, S., & Rubin, G. J. (2020). How to improve adherence with quarantine: Rapid review of the evidence. *Public Health, 182,* 163–169.

Weinstein, N., Vansteenkiste, M., & Paulmann, S. (2020). Don't you say it that way! Experimental evidence that controlling voices elicit defiance. *Journal of Experimental Social Psychology, 88,* 103949. https://doi.org/10.1016/j.jesp.201 9.103949

Wilder-Smith, A., & Freedman, D. O. (2020). Isolation, quarantine, social distancing and community containment: Pivotal role for old-style public health measures in the novel coronavirus (2019-nCoV) outbreak. *Journal of Travel Medicine, 27*(2). https://doi.org/10.1093/jtm/taaa020

Wormwood, J. B., Lynn, S. K., Barrett, L. F., & Quigley, K.S. (2016). Threat perception after the Boston marathon bombings: The effects of personal relevance and conceptual framing. *Cognition and Emotion, 30*(3), 539–549.

Zhai, Y., & Du, X. (2020). Mental health care for international Chinese students affected by the COVID-19 outbreak. *The Lancet: Psychiatry, 7,* e22. https://doi.org/10.1016/S2215-0366(20)30089-4

Chapter 4

Psychological Modelling: A Rational Public Approach

The first chapter examined psychological modelling linked specifically to subtle behaviour change messaging that encouraged the public to adopt practices, often cued by subtle signals in the settings they entered, to change the way they behaved. One articulation of this approach presumed that people can be "nudged" in the right direction to change their behaviour. This outcome can be achieved through messaging that encourages individuals to consider and weight up risks and benefits, but recognises that people may not be able to make objective and rationale judgements, and instead need to be steered towards specific decisions by having their perceptions of the world subtly manipulated through environmental cues. Change the beginning of this sentence: 'As Chapter Two showed, another approach is to focus another approach is to focus on the role and impact of social reference groups to which people turn for leadership or hints about how to behave in different settings.

Other psychological modelling has indicated that sometimes behaviour change can only be achieved through reasoned decision making on the part of members of the public. The process begins with messaging designed to shift a person's thoughts and feelings (i.e., beliefs and attitudes) about specific issues so as to establish a cognitive orientation towards them that will trigger internal motivation to change behaviour. A more conscious effort is required on the part of individuals in choosing to change their behaviour than was the case in a nudging scenario. People needed to believe that the behaviour change itself would deliver significant benefits (positive belief) and that it was the right thing to do (positive attitude).

Psychologists also discovered that while shifting people's beliefs and attitudes regarding a specific behaviour in the right direction was *necessary* to motivate behaviour change, it was not always *sufficient* to ensure it actually happened. Targeted individuals were also influenced in their behaviour change dispositions by their perceptions of whether other people were displaying the behaviour patterns they were being encouraged to adopt (known as "subjective norms") and whether they thought they were capable of making the behaviour change being encouraged (known as "behavioural control"). There are two theories that were significant in framing

DOI: 10.4324/9781003274308-4

how this process works: the theory of reasoned action and the theory of planned behaviour.

The theory of reasoned action model was built on the premise that people perform behaviour that is under their own control and based upon internal cognitive processes that determine the value of a behaviour to them (Ajzen & Fishbein, 1980; Fishbein & Ajzen, 1975). Action is deemed to be determined by reasoning through which individuals calculate the costs and benefits of specific behaviours. In other words, the model presumed that people think before they act. Specific behaviours were believed to result in specific outcomes that were, in turn, internally evaluated in advance. The theory of planned behaviour was an extension of the theory of reasoned action (Ajzen, 1991). The development of the second model recognised that not all behaviours are under an individual's personal control and that behaviour change depends upon whether people believe they *can* change.

A Reasoning Public

According to the theory of reasoned action, underlying each behavioural action is an *intention*. This is a reason or motive for performing the behaviour. The concept of intention implies that behaviour tends to be pre-planned. Even when we are doing something out of the ordinary, we may have planned ahead when we will do it and where. So, for instance, someone may have bought us a hot-air balloon ride as a birthday present. This is not something we would routinely do. Nonetheless, this particular experience is pre-organised with a specific supplier and a pre-specified time and requires us to travel to a pre-specified location.

Some behaviours, even ones that are not out of ordinary, can occur spontaneously, however, and so are not preceded by a previously reasoned intention. Closer inspection of the behaviour and when it occurred though might reveal that it is an action that we had thought about previously but without planning to perform at this particular moment. We might be walking past a shoe shop and see a pair of shoes we really like and decide in that moment to buy them. A generalised intention to upgrade our shoe wear was present in the back of our mind but was triggered in that moment by a serendipitous experience.

Accompanying the behaviour is an *attitude*. The attitude in this case refers to the behaviour itself and not an orientation towards the object of the behaviour. We may indeed think that the new pair of shoes will look good on us, but the performance of the purchase behaviour is grounded in the thought that it would be better to go into the shop in that moment rather than having to make special arrangements to come back to it later. Moreover, the desired shoes are there in front of us and if we pass up on this opportunity to buy them, someone else might come in later and buy them instead. Hence, that "in-the-moment" behaviour is favourably evaluated and this makes it more likely to occur.

An *attitude* is also closely linked to another internal concept, a *belief*. Beliefs comprise perceptions of likely outcomes of a behaviour. If buying a new pair of shoes is perceived as potentially beneficial because your existing shoes are getting worn out and you need to look good at work, then cognitively the scene is set for the purchase to be made. The spontaneous purchase might also be underpinned by the belief that it could be difficult to arrange another time specially to revisit the shop to make the purchase. Hence, beliefs and attitudes work together as cognitive precursors of behaviour.

Further perceptions, which can also be regarded broadly as beliefs, form a part of this predictive model concerning *subjective norms*. These are perceptions of the behaviour of other people and also of the assumed reactions of others to one's own behaviour (and its outcomes). These norms can be especially powerful when we perceive them to be held by people who are important to us or whose opinions are important to us. We make an assessment therefore about whether a behaviour will be seen as acceptable or expected by other people on the basis of how others generally behave or in terms of the feedback others have given us about our own behaviour or intentions. Of course, these "other" reference points for our behaviour may not always be available to us and then we are dependent upon our own internal reasoning.

Finally, there are other factors that play a part in the behaviour decision-making process. These *external variables* can be especially significant in persuasion scenarios where an outside agent is trying to get us to change our behaviour. The coronavirus lockdown scenario can be regarded as a multi-faceted persuasion programme designed to encourage people across the country to change their usual behaviour patterns.

These factors include personal characteristics of people such as their age, gender, socio-economic class, ethnicity, religion, sexual orientation, where they live, usual activity patterns, interests and hobbies, values and personality attributes. Other important external variables include their beliefs and attitudes concerning others, and especially those representing the agents seeking to achieve public behaviour change. The latter will include people's thoughts and feelings about politicians in general, political leaders, government institutions, medical and science experts and journalists and the media – in other words the key players behind the behaviour change programme, the collation of back-up evidence to support this programme, and those involved in reporting and analysing the actions of government and experts.

Persuasion Psychology and Behaviour Control

The original basic model of persuading people to change their behaviour focused on securing initial attitude change which was conceived to motivate eventual changes in behaviour. A group of communications experts at Yale University, led by Carl Hovland, developed a model for studying attitude and behaviour change persuasion starting with a basic premise of "who said what to whom" (Hovland et al., 1949, 1953). Within this framework therefore a number of distinct component parts were differentiated that included a *source* of a *message* that is sent via a specific *channel* to a target *audience*. It is necessary to analyse and understand the nature of the source, the message, the communication channel and the audience to determine whether a specific persuasion attempt will be successful with a specific target audience (Markova, 2008).

In the Yale framework, it is important that the *source* is perceived by the *audience* to be attractive and likeable, as having authority, credibility, competence and expertise, and integrity and trustworthiness. If the source scores well on these attributes (and other relevant evaluations), his or her persuasiveness is enhanced (Hovland & Weiss, 1951).

In the first instance, people are more likely to accept persuasive arguments from people they perceive as attractive (Chaiken, 1979). Audiences also look for characteristics in a source that they see in themselves. Perceived similarities between audiences and sources also encourage audiences to accept what a source tells them to think or to do (Goethals & Nelson, 1973).

Credibility is especially important for sources. Research has shown that sources regarded as credible are far more likely to command the respect of an audience and the things they say will be believed (O'Keefe, 2002). This criterion is especially critical in the context of government statements designed to get people to make radical behaviour changes in their everyday lives – a request many will not feel comfortable about or readily willing to comply with. Credibility derives in turn from perceived expertise which will derive from a preceding reputation, built upon their qualifications, experience and achievements. If these credentials all stack up convincingly, then audiences will have more confidence in sources and a greater inclination to comply with their behaviour change requests. An expert source is usually regarded as more trustworthy (Demidogen, 2010; O'Keefe, 2002).

If a *message* is to change a receiver's attitude and then their behaviour, it must be persuasive. This means it must contain specific ingredients according to which it will be judged by those on the receiving end. These *message* attributes represent a distinct set of assessment criteria from those used to evaluate the *source*.

The *channel* through which a message is received also determines the extent to which a *source* and *message* are persuasive. Channels include face-to-face conversation, a live event with one speaker addressing an audience or crowd, a theatrical performance, one-to-one and one-to-many written correspondence, an article in a publication, a broadcast on radio or television, and text, audio or video messages on web sites distributed over the internet. *Channels* can vary in their effectiveness which is determined by how they present information and the degree to which receivers in an audience engage with them. Some channels are also more trusted than others by receivers.

Messages might also be presented along with other messages. The order of presentation can make a difference to the impact of any one message. Messages presented at the beginning or end of a sequence tend to be the most memorable afterwards (Haugtvedt & Wegener, 1994). Within a message itself, one theory that surfaced was that the narrative should build to a climax at the end when the key argument becomes fully presented, although the benefits of this approach could often be quite small (O'Keefe, 2002).

Another structural feature of persuasive messages is whether they present one-sided arguments or two-sided arguments. In the first case, the message argues a position from a single perspective. Persuasive messages will usually try to convince an audience to shift their attitudes or behaviour in a specific direction by giving a reason for doing so. There may be counter-arguments for not doing so, but in one-sided messages, these alternative positions are ignored. In two-sided messages, alternative perspectives might be presented and critiqued. Hence, in a campaign to get people to stop smoking, the message may focus on the harmful health side effects of this behaviour. Counter-argument might be presented that these side effects are not experienced by all smokers or the smoker may site an example of an elderly relative who has smoked all his life without ill effects.

In two-sided messages these defences against the initial persuasive messages to stop smoking might also be examined and then dismantled by showing that the elderly relative who had smoked for many years, was lucky and that in many more cases, smokers die earlier or experience health problems in later years that undermine their quality of life. One-sided messages have been found to work well on people who are less knowledgeable about the issues and less likely to challenge the argument being put forward. For more critical audiences that have already considered other points of view or who know the facts, two-sided messages can be more effective if they effectively dismantle the typical counter-arguments that audiences might be expected to put forward as defences (Hovland et al., 1949; Larson, 1992).

The depth to which the arguments in a message are processed will therefore be driven by the character of the message itself and whether it is designed to trigger cognitive or emotional reactions in the audience and also the orientation of the audience towards the issues being presented. The psychological responses to messages are not triggered simply by whether they contain one-sided or two-sided arguments but also by whether the arguments represent a central aspect of the message or not for members of the audience (Chaiken & Eagly, 1976).

All these message attributes are important for creating effective rational appeals to change behaviour. In the case of a pandemic caused by a new virus for which no vaccine protection exists, the significance of physical or social distancing measures can be regarded as a rational argument on the grounds that the virus is mainly airborne and that it makes sense therefore to keep people physically apart as much as possible to halt its spread. Yet, the case being made here requires the audience, in this case the public, to make far-reaching changes to their normal behaviour. This request goes far beyond seeking to change one specific behaviour such as smoking or alcohol consumption or wearing seatbelts. Publics around the world were asked to tolerate fundamental lifestyle changes for an indefinite period.

No matter how rationally persuasive was the initial messaging about the coronavirus and about how to slow down accelerating rates of infection, many people could still be expected to produce counter-arguments given the magnitude of the behaviours changes being demanded of them. In this case, the persuasive messaging needed to be bolstered with strong internal beliefs (based on risk) and equally strong emotional appeals (based on fear) to motivate the targeted behaviour change.

Fear has been a commonly used internal motivator of behaviour change for many years (Petty & Cacioppo, 1986; Stiff, 1993). It is essential to establish an optimal level of it, however, to achieve the desired results. A certain degree of fear arousal in the audience can heighten their attention to a message. Over-playing the fear, however, can disrupt rational message processing. Moreover, the fear factor must fit the occasion and have relevance to the final objective. Exaggeration of fear, if identified by the audience, could diminish message and source credibility (Boster & Mongeau, 1984). Further, it is important to be sensitive to the emotional condition of the audience. Low fear appeals work much better than high fear appeals with people who are already anxious (Goldstein, 1959). Anxious people might be less capable psychologically if coping with extreme threat compared with more emotionally stable people.

Pre-specified *audiences* are the eventual targets in terms of attitude and behaviour change. In the case of the COVID-19 pandemic, the "audience" was everybody. Persuasive communications tend to be designed with specific audiences in mind. Audiences must be attentive to messages if they are effectively to absorb what they say. Unless they do this, messages are unlikely to have much impact.

The general intelligence and knowledgeability of audiences in regard to the subject matter of a persuasive message are important mediating factors that can render messages more or less persuasive with particular receivers. Audiences evaluate sources and messages by adopting their own benchmarks for specific evaluative criteria such as source credibility and message accuracy.

The familiarity of audiences with subject matter will also determine the way in which they process incoming messages. As we will see, according to dual-process theories, audiences are influenced by making sense of messages either by picking apart their arguments and critiquing their accuracy or by judging how attractive the message or source appears to be. One approach involves a deeper level of processing than the other (Petty & Wegener, 1999).

Persuasion Theory: Elaboration Likelihood Model

One of the widest used models to investigate and explain the process of persuasion in relation to changes in people's attitudes is the elaboration-likelihood model. It was developed by Richard E. Petty and John T. Cacioppo and has been used by many other persuasion researchers. Their focus was placed on developing reliable and valid explanations of how people's attitudes might be changed by specific information campaigns (Petty & Cacioppo, 1986). Campaign messages would be produced for communication to people perhaps via direct, face-to-face, conversations or more often through mediated channels such as media advertising.

The model has also been described as a "dual-process" theory because it combines two principal elements. Its basic premise is that when people are presented with messages designed to change the way they think and feel about something – whether this is an issue, an institution, another person, or a commercial brand – there are two major pathways that are deployed in this process. These have been called the central route and the peripheral route to persuasion. The central route involves the individual examining the message really carefully for its core arguments and the information it provides concerning the object or issue about which it is seeking to change people's attitudes. The peripheral route to persuasion involves making a much more superficial or simpler judgement about the message based on who is sending it, what it looks like and whether the person receiving it likes the way it presents its message (Petty et al., 1983).

In an advertisement for a new vacuum cleaner, for example, central processing would entail assessing how functionally effective it is at cleaning different surfaces, how easy it might be to service, and whether it is light and easy to move around. A peripheral assessment might be made more on the basis of how the product looks, whether it is demonstrated by an attractive actor or model, whether there is humour in it, or whether it, in the case of television advertising, is accompanied by appealing background music. It might also have been recommended by a celebrity who is well-liked, even though they may have no specialist expertise in the way vacuum cleaners work.

Both central processing and peripheral processing can represent effective routes to persuasion under the right conditions. With relatively inexpensive items, peripheral processing could become relatively more important because such items might not be regarded as worth the effort of central processing. With more expensive items, however, the reverse could be true. "Expensive" in this context might not be evaluated simply in monetary terms. It might also refer to the cost incurred by an individual in taking the message seriously or not. An example would be a persuasive message concerned with changing people's attitudes and behaviours in a national health emergency where the cost is their personal safety.

When getting people to change their mindset, often as a precursor to getting them to change their behaviour, a persuasive message must do more than simply pass on information about the need for change. Its "persuasiveness" derives from its ability to trigger the idea for change and energise the motivation in the individual to actually change. A starting point to this chain of processes is that the message must initially interest the recipient. Dry rational or empirical messaging – the fuel of central processing – might not be enough. The message needs to be dressed up in its style of presentation to incorporate energy and pace, and also relevance to those at whom it is targeted. It must engage them cognitively so that they weigh up the importance of the message's information to their own lives and needs. It must also engage them emotionally so that they *feel* the need to change (Morris et al., 2005).

As indicated by the concept of 'psychological reactance' message recipients, message recipients must not only believe the message and perceive its relevance and usefulness (cognitive central processing) and feel (an emotional attitudinal response) that they would find the change being encouraged personally pleasurable or beneficial, they must also feel that the ultimate choice is theirs (a matter of personal control). If the individual develops a strong negative feeling about the messages themselves and the change to their behaviour it advocates and if they believe they are being railroaded into it, there will be resistance to respond in the way the message sender hopes for. Instead of a compliance response, there will be a boomerang effect (Griffin, 2013).

Some messages can be highly effective at shifting public attitudes and behaviour even when their subject matter holds little interest for most people. The application of the peripheral route to persuasion can be helpful in this context. People end up making judgements about the object or issue under consideration on the basis of very general impressions about it. If they are being asked to consider how to vote for a political candidate, for example, they might, of course, evaluate that individual on the basis of the policies for which they stand or believe in, or whether they display good values through the things they say or do, or simply on the basis of how they look and sound.

The source of the message, and its credibility and likeability, are other factors that come into play in the persuasion process and can bolster a message even when its arguments are not as compelling or convincing as they could be (Booth-Butterfield & Gutowski, 1993). An effective source can drive forward specific arguments and motivate recipients to process them (and even be persuaded by them). Strong messages and/or messages that are stylistically presented can be persuasive (Mosler, 2006).

Increasingly, online platforms such as social networking sites have come to play an influential role in persuasion processes. Here, elaborate arguments in favour of an object or issue can be articulated with endorsements from credible sources including original sources, authority figures and ordinary people, to create a highly influential setting with which message recipients can become deeply psychologically engaged (Ott et al., 2016; Wu et al., 2011).

There are also opportunities in these settings to repeat messages many times. Whereas a single exposure to a message designed to influence recipients' behaviour might be insufficient to have much impact, several exposures can build up a cumulative effect that is more powerful once those on the receiving end have been given the chance to consider persuasive appeals in more detail (Cacioppo & Petty, 1989). The message processing might be "central" and "peripheral" in nature. Where a central processing strategy might leave recipients unconvinced by core arguments for behaviour change, other stylistic features such as the attractiveness of the message source or appeals to the consciences of recipients to accept a decision that has a wider "good" at heart could sway them to change their behaviour nonetheless.

Another aspect of weighing up messages in times of crisis is to consider "personal" and "other" risks of specific courses of action or of failing to take them. Objective risks calculations could be difficult where there are insufficient data to base them upon (e.g., chances of dying from a highly infectious disease with and without specific interventionist behaviour changes), so then we must rely instead on whatever examples of possible outcomes come most readily to mind. People therefore frequently use what have been called "mental shortcuts" to making up their minds about objects, people or issues (Kahneman, 2003). As we saw in the discussion of nudging, these shortcuts have also been referred to as "heuristics".

When using heuristic assessments, we rely on personal judgements about the quality of the message source rather than the quality of the message. Is the source delivering the message likeable? Do we feel we can trust them? Do they seem to have authority? Do they seem to have relevant expertise? As our opinion about the message source improves, so our inclination to believe, accept and act upon what they tell us also strengthens (Cialdini, 2001). In the COVID-19 pandemic, the principal source was the government, backed up by associated medical and scientific experts carefully selected by government. Trust in government and those working directly with it was therefore going to be important to public engagement and compliance with behaviour change messages.

From Reasoned Action to Planned Behaviour

The theory of reasoned action accumulated a lot of empirical support as a predictor of behavioural outcomes across a wide range of settings. An analysis of internal beliefs and attitudes concerning a specific behaviour and about the behaviour and behavioural norms of others can produce accurate predictions of the way a specific individual will behave in response to someone urging them to behave in that way (Albarracín et al., 2001; Hagger et al., 2002).

Research into persuasion and behaviour change revealed, however, that the reasoned action model's variables were insufficient to account effectively for how people do eventual behave. Behaviour change can occur if our beliefs and attitudes about specific behaviours and our perceptions of how others behave or are likely to react to particular types of behaviour change. These internal cognitive factors can predict and explain behaviour change, but not always. When failure occurs, it was often found to be explained by a perceived inability on the part of individuals to countenance or be capable of making a specific change to their behaviour (Ajzen, 1991). This last point led to the emergence of the theory of planned behaviour from the theory of reasoned action.

According to this theory, behaviour is shaped by three principal factors: attitudes, subjective norms and perceived behavioural control. Together these factors can work together to create an intention to behave in a particular way. This is a motivational component that drives eventual overt behaviour. Intention in turn triggers a behavioural outcome. This might represent a continuation of established behaviour or a change to behaviour or the adoption of a completely new behaviour.

In this setting, attitude refers to internal thoughts and feelings a person might have about a specific behaviour. If performing specific behaviour is believed to lead to some kind of reward or benefit in the form of a pleasurable end-result or enhanced quality of life, then a positive attitude will form about it. If, however, a behaviour that a person is being encouraged to adopt holds no obvious value for them and they cannot envisage how it might benefit them, their thoughts and feelings about it might be relatively neutral or even negative if performing it is regarded as an inconvenience or nuisance.

Subjective norms refer to a person's recognition or awareness of what others in their social circle or wider society think and feel about the target behaviour and more importantly how they behave as well. If a health campaign is designed to get specific individuals to change their behaviour or adopt new behaviour, seeing others around them willingly adopting this behaviour and also speaking positively about it will create a positive climate of opinion and action around the behaviour that will encourage the person being targeted to follow suit. If others reject that behaviour or simply exhibit little interest in it, the environmental conditions will not be created that encourage the person to change their own habits.

Perceived behavioural controls represent judgements a person makes about whether they would be able to change their behaviour in the way a campaign or persuader would like them to. A campaign might try to persuade overweight people to lose weight by changing their eating habits or by taking more exercise. If the individual feels unable to go along with these changes, even though they may know it would be good for them and others are encouraging them to do it as well, the chances of behaviour change will be diminished.

Intentions are linked to an internal desire to change or adopt new behaviour. Holding positive attitudes towards a behaviour and recognising that others believe in this behaviour and perform it, and knowing that adoption of the behaviour is within their grasp and ability, leads to an internal drive to perform the behaviour. This might be accompanied also by a cognitive component in which the person plans out how they will go about changing their behaviour.

Health behaviour specialists have utilised the theory of planned behaviour as a theoretical basis for behaviour change exercises. In these studies, people targeted for change have their attitudes and beliefs shaped by environmental stimuli, often in the form of informational messages or emotional stimulation designed to manipulate their attitudes towards the target behaviour and its intended outcomes and their beliefs about whether this behaviour or widely received by others (especially those of social importance to target persons) and their beliefs that this change to their behaviour is something of which they are well capable.

In an examination of the findings of studies of behaviour change linked to alcohol consumption and diet, the predictive value of this theory was confirmed by much of the evidence. In other words, targeted behaviour change was more likely to occur when relevant attitudes and beliefs were effectively constructed and lined up to increase motivation or intention to change (Hagger et al., 2016; McMillan & Conner, 2003).

These two theories represented gradually evolving thinking among psychologists about how thoughts, feelings and behaviours are inter-linked which had been taking place since the 1950s (Fishbein & Ajzen, 1975). Initial thinking, under the auspices of the theory of reasoned action was that if we want to persuade people to change their behaviour, it helps if they have a positive *attitude* (i.e., feeling) towards that behaviour. It also helps if they perceive that other people want them to adopt this behaviour, a concept called a *subjective norm*. If their attitude towards a behaviour is positive and they believe others expect them to behave this way, this creates a motivational state in which they develop an *intention* to adopt the desired behaviour (Sheppard et al., 1988).

The emergence of research shows that developing an intention to behave a specific way does not always successfully translate in the adoption of that behaviour. The relationship between behavioural intention and overt behaviour cannot be taken for granted (Norberg et al., 2007). One reason why this occurs is that with some behaviours, their eventual performance could lie beyond the control of the individual. A person might be persuaded in principle to adopt a specific pattern of behaviour and is both favourably disposed towards doing so and believes it would be a good idea, in the end they simply cannot bring themselves to do it. This realisation led to the development of a new factor called perceived *behavioural control*.

There was also a further component to this factor and that was the belief that a behaviour could be performed successfully. People need to perceive that they have the control to make a specific behaviour happen that someone else is persuading them to adopt. In this context, it is important for people to hold an intrinsic belief they have the ability to perform that behaviour and that it is not beyond them.

Hence, a promotional campaign might try to persuade people to buy a particular brand of car, but then an individual who was potentially in the market for the car loses their job and simply cannot afford to make the purchase, so they don't. In a different scenario, the same person might get a new job and then becomes technically able to afford to buy that car, but their earlier job loss has left them feeling insecure to a point where they believe it is high risk to make that kind of financial outlay even though at that moment they can afford to do so. In some instances, therefore, loss of control over a behaviour occurs because the individual believes they cannot perform it and, in other instances, for explicit objective reasons (e.g., they cannot afford to keep buying hand sanitiser). In other cases, it is a matter of subjective perception, whereby they could perform the behaviour if they really wanted to but believe they cannot (e.g., belief they cannot work from home when with some adjustments they could).

In the theory of planned behaviour, therefore, the concept of *control beliefs* is added to the other factors from the theory of reasoned action. These beliefs may have been learned from past personal experiences or from the second-hand experiences of others the person knows and trusts. The importance of perceived control over behaviour change on the part of the individual has been confirmed empirically by studies across a range of behaviour change settings (Armitage & Conner, 2001; Hagger et al., 2002; McEachen et al., 2011).

The theory of planned behaviour has not gone unchallenged. Some critics argue that it provides an incomplete model for predicting behavioural outcomes. There are other variables that are important and need to be taken into account when analysing whether a behaviour change will prove to be effective. In the next chapter, a broader-based theoretical model is examined that incorporates other potential predictor variables for behaviour over and above those outlined in the panned model. The criticisms are informative and offer ideas about further psychological variables we might take into account when trying to predict and explain whether people will or will not comply with specific behaviour change requests. They do not invalidate the predictive and explanatory usefulness of the variables already included in the model however (Kan & Fabrigar, 2017).

Research has shown that future behaviour patterns can be strongly influenced by past habits, moral obligations and personal identity with the behaviour change being sought or encouraged (Bentler & Speckart, 1979; Biddle et al., 1987; Ouellette & Wood, 1998; Schwartz &Tessler, 1972). Human behaviour also develops over time through the formation of habits. Specific behaviour patterns become established in particular settings that are regarded as the normal or expected way to behave or that represent effective behaviours in those situations as learned through trial and error (Wood & Neal, 2007, 2009; Wood et al., 2014).

One further area of debate concerns where spontaneous behaviour might fit in which for some psychologists represents the explanatory "Achilles' heel" of the theory of planned behaviour which focuses on explaining rationally determined action. Such deliberate action has been conceived to depend upon a person having the motivation and opportunity to perform a behaviour. These two elements are crucial in creating the behavioural intention or internal motivation that ultimately drives the person to perform a specific behaviour or to change their behaviour in some way when being persuaded to do this. When motivation and opportunity are absent, a specific behaviour might still occur if the person holds a positive attitude towards performing it, believes others would expect this behaviour or have encouraged the person to perform it, and the individual feels able to perform it (Fazio, 1986; Fazio & Olson, 2014).

Moving on to the COVID-19 pandemic and the government's attempts to introduce interventions in the form of behavioural restrictions, success will depend on a number of factors according to the theory of planned behaviour. These comprise:

perceptions that a specific course of action will be effective in achieving specific objectives (Behaviour-Related Beliefs);

the evaluation that it is the right thing to do (Behaviour-Related Attitude);

perceptions that people in general are compliant with the need for the outlined behaviour change (Normative Beliefs);

the perception that personally important reference groups (e.g., family and close friends) are on board (Subjective Norms);

perceptions that there will be external support to help them through troubling times (Control Beliefs);

and, finally, the view that the behaviour changes being requested will be feasible or viable for them (Perceived Behavioural Control).

If all these predictor variables line together in a consistent way, then the likelihood of public compliance with behaviour change will be enhanced. If any of these cognitive dispositions are negative rather than positive then public compliance will be weaker.

The Challenges to Compliance

The imposition of a lockdown on normal life could only be successful if people complied with its restrictions. The success of this type of intervention will be manifest in how people behave. They might not like the lockdown – and so hold negative attitudes towards it – but despite this ill-feeling they still follow the new rules of behaviour because they have been persuaded that this is what they need to do. Hence, despite the development of psychological models of persuasion which examine the significance of cognitive variables such as beliefs and attitudes in relation to behaviour change, behaviour can change even though internal judgements about this change remain negative.

There were concerns that the draconian restrictions of full societal lockdown were met with public resistance. Psychologists are familiar with the concept of "psychological reactance" whereby people reject attempts to constrain their freedom of choice in the way they behave as a matter of principle (Brehm, 1966, 1972; Brehm & Brehm, 1981). The strength of reactance depends upon the importance of the freedoms being removed and the stringency with which this is done (Steindl et al., 2015). There are also known to be variances between different cultures in the degree to which they are willing to accept such restrictions on their behaviour. Eastern collectivistic cultures are generally more compliant to collective authority than are Western individualistic cultures (Iyengar & Lepper, 1999).

Another concern was that there would be "wear out" of compliance after a fairly short period of time. The greater the degree of restriction over everyday behaviour, the sooner this effect would be felt. This is a concept derived from marketing and recognises that specific promotional messages can lose their ability to persuade people to adopt or change a specific behaviour after repeated exposure (Danaher, 1996; East, 2003). Throughout the first pandemic lockdown in the UK and beyond, national and provincial government briefings provided constant reminders of the need to "stay home" or "protect the NHS" or "keep their social distance" from others. It is not simply the passage of time that matters here. Of further significance is the optimal spacing of persuasive messages over time to keep them fresh (Bass et al., 2007).

Compliance under these circumstances depends on other conditions being in place. People are more likely to change their behaviour voluntarily despite not being pleased about it if they are persuaded by rational arguments showing that it is our best interests to change. They will comply more willingly if the message for change comes from a source they know and trust. People will change their behaviour if they are gradually encouraged to do so in small steps. Initially, they might be persuaded to make a small change and then having got that far, they become more susceptible to the influence of requests for further and more pronounced behaviour changes. They might also be more likely to change their behaviour if others are doing likewise and they wish to be consistent with them (Cialdini & Goldstein, 2004).

In the context of the coronavirus pandemic, the government's non-pharmaceutical interventions required people to limit their outdoor behaviour. While they were allowed to go out to shop for essentials, even then they were advised to restrict these trips as much as they could. Evidence emerged from early lockdown research with the public that significant minorities of people (39%) envisaged shopping more often than this because they wanted to avoid queues Despite people being warned to avoid visiting elderly relatives, there remained a few people (10%) that felt they simply could not comply with this advice because of the immediate needs of their relatives (King's College London, 2020).

These responses however were probably less connected to reactance or wearout than to rational judgements about what people felt they could or could not reasonably go along with. Many people, of course complied fully at the outset, and others not so much. Although some members of the public might have felt that the restrictions were not pleasant or easy, they could be persuaded to comply if they thought that the measures would be effective, were the right thing to do, that others were complying and, with some adjustments, they were able to take sufficient control of necessary life adjustments to comply.

Pros and Cons of Planned Behaviour Modelling of COVID Compliance

To work effectively, messaging about interventions to mitigate the chances of being infected with COVID-19 needed to engage people sufficiently and appropriately to shift their attitudes and beliefs in the right direction to motivate compliance with behavioural restrictions. Much attention was given during the 2020 coronavirus pandemic to the modelling of epidemiologists, but this work had little value in terms of modelling whether there would be compliance with lockdown restrictions. Hindsight, based on awareness and analysis of behaviour change and control in past pandemics, indicates that psychological modelling could be highly relevant in the context of judging the kinds of interventions that might prove effective in controlling virus transmission in the pandemic that swept across the world in 2020.

Research with people in The Netherlands concerning public perceptions of the influenza A (H1N1) pandemic in 2009 found that people's confidence that they knew how to protect themselves from this disease, intention to comply with preventive measures and perceived severity of the disease decreased as their knowledge about the new disease improved (Bults et al., 2011).

Over the first few months of the outbreak public anxiety levels rose and then stabilised. People who were most strongly inclined to adopt preventive measures also were the ones who perceived the new disease as more serious. Higher disease-related anxiety and stronger belief in their ability to protect themselves from infection were also linked with greater adoption of preventive measures. These findings were consistent with what might have been predicted by the theory of planned behaviour for which perceived behavioural control was a crucial factor in motivating the adoption of protective behaviour change. Later chapters will revisit the theory of planned behaviour to review its efficacy as a foundational model underpinning pandemic control strategy in relation to interventions such as physical distancing, personal protective measures and vaccination.

References

Ajzen, I. (1991). The theory of planned behavior. *Organizational Behavior and Human Decision Processes*, 50(2), 179–211.

Ajzen, I., & Fishbein, M. (1980). *Understanding Attitudes and Predicting Social Behavior*. Englewood-Cliffs, NJ: Prentice-Hall.

Albarracín, D., Johnson, B. T., Fishbein, M., & Muellerleile, P. A. (2001). Theories of reasoned action and planned behavior as models of condom use: A meta-analysis. *Psychological Bulletin*, 127(1), 142–161.

Armitage, C. J., & Conner, M. (2001). Efficacy of the theory of planned behaviour: A meta-analytic review. *British Journal of Social Psychology*, 40(4), 471–499.

Bass, F. M., Norris, B., Majumdar, S., & Mirthi, B. P. S. (2007). Wearout effects of different advertising themes: A dynamic Bayesian model of the advertising – sales relationship. *Marketing Science*, 26(2), 179–195.

Bentler, P. M., & Speckart, G. (1979). Models of attitude – behavior relations. *Psychological Review*, 86(5), 452–464.

Biddle, B., Bank, B., & Slavings, R. (1987). Norms, preferences, identities and retention decisions. *Social Psychology Quarterly*, 50(4), 322–337.

Booth-Butterfield, S., & Gutowski, C. (1993). Message modality and source credibility can interact to affect argument processing. *Communication Quarterly*, 41(1), 77–89.

Boster, F. J., & Mongeau, P. (1984). Fear-arousing persuasive messages. *Communication Yearbook*, 8, 330–375.

Brehm, J. W. (1966). *A Theory of Psychological Reactance*. New York, NY: Academic Press.

Brehm, J. W. (1972). *Responses to Loss of Freedom: A Theory of Psychological Reactance*. Morristown, NJ: General Learning Corporation.

Brehm, J. W., & Brehm, S. S. (1981). *Psychological Reactance: A Theory of Freedom and Control*. New York, NY: Academic Press.

Bults, M., Beaujean, D. J., de Zwart, O., Kok, G., van Empelen, P., van Steenbergen, J. E., Richardus, J. H., & Voeten, H. A. (2011). Perceived risk, anxiety, and behavioural responses of the general public during the early phase of the Influenza A (H1N1) pandemic in the Netherlands: results of three consecutive online surveys. *BMC Public Health*, 3(11), 2. https://doi.org/10.1186/1471-2458-11-2

Cacioppo, J. T., & Petty, R. E. (1989). Effects of message repetition on argument processing, recall and persuasion. *Basic and Applied Social Psychology*, 10(1), 3–12.

Chaiken, S. (1979). Communicator physical attractiveness and persuasion. *Journal of Personality and Social Psychology*, 37(8), 1387–1397.

Chaiken, S., & Eagly, A. H. (1976). Communication modality as a determinant of message comprehensibility. *Journal of Personality and Social Psychology*, 34, 605–614.

Cialdini, R. B. (2001). *Influence: Science and Practice* (4th ed.). Boston, MA: Allyn & Bacon.

Cialdini, R. B., & Goldstein, N. J. (2004). Compliance and conformity. *Annual Review of Psychology*, 55, 591–621.

Danaher, P. (1996). Wearout effects in target marketing. *Marketing Letters*, 7(3), 275–287.

Demidogen, U. D. (2010). The roots of research in (political) persuasion: Ethos, pathos, logos and the Yale studies of persuasive communication. *Journal of Social Inquiry*, 3(1), 189–201.

East, R. (2003). Wearout, carryover effects and decay of advertising. In *The Effect of Advertising and Display* (pp. 23–47). Boston, MA: Springer.

Fazio, R. H. (1986). How do attitudes guide behavior? *Handbook of Motivation and Cognition: Foundations of Social Behavior* (pp. 204–243). New York, NY: Guilford Press.

Fazio, R. H., & Olson, M. A. (2014). The MODE model: Attitude-behavior processes as a function of motivation and opportunity. In J. W. Sherman, B. Gawronski, & Y. Trope (Eds.), *Dual Process Theories of the Social Mind* (pp. 155–171). New York, NY: Guilford Press.

Fishbein, M., & Ajzen, I. (1975). *Belief, Attitude, Intention, and Behavior: An Introduction to Theory and Research*. San Francisco, CA: Addison-Wesley.

Goethals, G. R., & Nelson, R. E. (1973). Similarity in the influence process: The belief/value distinction. *Journal of Personality and Social Psychology*, 25, 117–122.

Goldstein, M. J. (1959). The relationship between coping and avoiding behaviour and response to fear-arousing propaganda. *Journal of Abnormal and Social Psychology*, 58, 247–257.

Griffin, L. K. (2013). Narrative, truth and trial. *The Georgetown Law Journal*, 101, 281–335.

Hagger, M. S., Chan, D. K. C., Protogerou, C., & Chatzisarantis, N. L. D. (2016). Using meta-analytic path analysis to test theoretical predictions in health behavior: An illustration based on meta-analyses of the theory of planned behavior. *Preventive Medicine*, 89, 154–161.

Hagger, M. S., Chatzisarantis, N. L. D., & Biddle, S. J. H. (2002). A meta-analytic review of the theories of reasoned action and planned behavior in physical activity: Predictive validity and the contribution of additional variables. *Journal of Sport & Exercise Psychology, 24*(1), 3–32.

Haugtvedt, C. P., & Wegener, D. T. (1994). Message order effects in persuasion: An attitude strength perspective. *Journal of Consumer Research, 21*, 205. https://doi.org/10.1086/209393

Hovland, C. I., Janis, I. L., & Kelley, H. H. (1953). *Communication and Persuasion: Psychological Studies of Opinion Change.* New Haven, CT: Yale University Press.

Hovland, C. I., Lumsdaine, A. A., & Sheffield, F. D. (1949). *Experiments on Mass Communication.* Princeton, NJ: Princeton University Press.

Hovland, C. I., & Weiss, W. (1951). The influence of source credibility on communication effectiveness. *Public Opinion Quarterly, 15*(4), 635–650.

Iyengar, S. S., & Lepper, M. R. (1999). Rethinking the value of choice: A cultural perspective on intrinsic motivation. *Journal of Personality and Social Psychology, 76*(3), 349–366.

Kahneman, D. (2003). A perspective on judgment and choice: Mapping bounded rationality. *American Psychologist, 58*, 697–720.

Kan, M., & Fabrigar, L. (2017). Theory of planned behaviour. *Encyclopedia of Personality and Individual Differences,* pp. 1–8. https://doi.org/10.1007/978-3-319-28099-8

King's College London (2020, 9th April). Life under lockdown: Coronavirus in the UK. Available at: https://www.kcl.ac.uk/news/life-under-lockdown-coronavirus-in-the-uk

Larson, C. U. (1992). *Persuasion: Reception and Responsibility.* Belmont, CA: Wadsworth.

Markova, I. (2008). Persuasion and social psychology. *Diogenes, 55*(1), 5–8.

McEachen, R. R., Conner, M., Taylor, N. J., & Lawton, R. J. (2011). Prospective prediction of health-related behaviours with the theory of planned behaviour: A meta-analysis. *Health Psychology Review, 5*(2), 97–144.

McMillan, B., & Conner, M. (2003). Using the theory of planned behaviour to understand alcohol and tobacco use in students. *Psychology, Health and Medicine, 8*(3), 317–328.

Morris, J. D., Singh, A. J., & Woo, C. (2005). Elaboration likelihood model: A missing intrinsic emotional implication. *Journal of Targeting, Measurement and Analysis for Marketing, 14*, 79–98.

Mosler, H.-J. (2006). Better be convincing or better be stylish? A theory based multi-agent simulation to explain minority influence in groups via arguments or via peripheral cues. *Journal of Artificial Societies and Social Simulation, 9*(3). https://www.jasss.org/9/3/4.html

Norberg, P. A., Horne, D. R., & Horne, D. A. (2007). The privacy paradox: Personal information disclosure intentions versus behaviors. *Journal of Consumer Affairs, 41*(1), 100–126.

O'Keefe, D. J. (2002). *Persuasion: Theory and Research.* Thousand Oaks, CA: SAGE Publications.

Ott, H. K., Vafeiadis, M., Kumble, S., & Waddell, T. F. (2016). Effect of message interactivity on product attitudes and purchase intentions. *Journal of Promotion Management, 22*(1), 89–106.

Ouellette, J. A., & Wood, W. (1998). Habit and intention in everyday life: The multiple processes by which past behavior predicts future behavior. *Psychological Bulletin*, 124(1), 54–74.

Petty, R. E., & Cacioppo, J. T. (1986). The elaboration likelihood model of persuasion. In L. Berkowitz (Ed.), *Advances in Experimental Social Psychology* (Vol. 19, pp. 123–205). New York, NY: Academic Press

Petty, R. E., Cacioppo, J. T., & Schumann, D. (1983). Central and peripheral routes to advertising effectiveness: The moderating role of involvement. *Journal of Consumer Research*, 10(2), 135–146.

Petty, R. E., & Wegener, D. T. (1999). The elaboration likelihood model: Current status and controversies. In S. Chaiken & Y. Trope (Eds.), *Dual Process Theories in Social Psychology* (pp. 37–72). New York, NY: Guilford Press.

Schwartz, S. H., & Tessler, R. C. (1972). A test of a model for reducing measured attitude-behavior discrepancies. *Journal of Personality and Social Psychology*, 24(2), 225–236.

Sheppard, B., Hartwick, J., & Warshaw, P. (1988). The theory of reasoned action: A meta-analysis of past research with recommendations for modifications and future research. *Journal of Consumer Research*, 15(3), 325–343.

Steindl, C., Jonas, E., Sittenthaler, S., Traut-Mattausch, E., & Greenberg, J. (2015). Understanding psychological reactance: New developments and findings. *Zeitschrift fur Psychologie*, 223(4), 205–214. https://doi.org/10.1027/2151-2 604/a000222

Stiff, J. B. (1993). *Persuasive Communication*. New York: Guilford.

Wood, W., Labrecque, J. S., Lin, P. Y., & Rünger, D. (2014). Habits in dual process models. In J. W. Sherman, B. Gawronski, & Y. Trope (Eds.), *Dual Process Theories of the Social Mind* (pp. 371–385). New York, NY: Guilford Press.

Wood, W., & Neal, D. T. (2007). A new look at habits and the habit-goal interface. *Psychological Review*, 114(4), 843–863.

Wood, W., & Neal, D. T. (2009). The habitual consumer. *Journal of Consumer Psychology*, 19(4), 579–592.

Wu, Y., Wong, J., Deng, Y., & Chang, K. (2011). An exploration of social media in public opinion convergence: Elaboration likelihood and semantic networks on political events. *2011 IEEE Ninth International Conference on dependable Autonomic and Secure Computing*, pp. 903–910. https://doi.org/10.11 09.DASC.2011.151

Chapter 5

Psychological Modelling: COM-B – A Custom-Built Theory

The effective implementation of interventions based on restricting people's movements and interpersonal interactions with others is reliant on public compliance. In addition to the lessons learned from earlier pandemics, further insights could be gleaned from the effectiveness of public health campaigns that were targeted at specific types of behaviour change linked to people's well-being, such as giving up tobacco smoking, drinking less alcohol, and changes to dietary habits. Nudging, social identity/group processes and planned behaviour change approaches were adopted in some of these instances to guide the way health campaigns were designed and their impact measured and to provide explanations of their overall effectiveness (Institute for Government, 2010).

When dealing with any of these cases, the extant understanding indicated that multiple measures were usually needed to achieve success. With a public health challenge on the scale of the COVID-19 pandemic, the need for a multi-faceted approach to bring it under control was probably an understatement. There were so many settings in which people might interact with others and hence become infected by this mostly airborne new virus, that only by closing down those spaces and encouraging people not to go out and intermingle could the pandemic be controlled. People around the world were told to stay at home. Leaving the home was then restricted to specified purposes and only under strict conditions. To achieve these outcomes, coordinated sets of restrictions were needed. These had to be deployed comprehensively and in a timely fashion (Mansdorf, 2020).

Moving beyond these models, other psychologists have identified additional variables and combinations of variables that might make a difference to whether people will comply with restrictions imposed from above on their behaviour. The nudge, group processes/social identity and planed behaviour models had demonstrated that they have some explanatory value in relation to pandemic behaviour restrictions and adoption of protective behaviours. These models, however, tended to confine their theorising around specific sets of factors. A widespread scan of psychological research, however, can reveal other predictors of this behaviour. Indeed, there could

DOI: 10.4324/9781003274308-5

be benefits for understanding to be gained from sometimes combining predictor variables from nudge theory and planned behaviour theory and then also from other theories.

While having theory is important in any research to provide explanation of relationships between variables and then to be able to forecast an event's consequences or outcomes, single theoretical models might be too narrowly definitive of key variables and choices in the context of major crises. In the case of pandemics, and especially one that affected the entire world on the scale of COVID-19, some experts have advised that a wider approach might be advisable in trying to understand how to tackle such events (Bish & Michie, 2010). By taking this approach, evidence will be considered from a broader pool of research.

In effect, Bish and Michie (2010) recommended the integration of different models that had previously been found to offer some relevance to the systematic of pandemics. Where a large-scale event necessitated extensive and diverse public behaviour changes, achievement of this outcome was likely to depend upon the application of a wide range of interventions. Not only did each of these interventions need to be effective in producing a specific change to people's behaviour patterns (e.g., making a point of keeping physically apart), when more than one intervention was used in combination with others, there needed to be some certainty that they would work effectively together. The last thing anyone would want if that the impact of one intervention counteracts or neutralises the impact of another.

Changing behaviour also usually requires earlier changes to internal psychological constructs such as attitudes, beliefs, perceptions and motivations. They might also depend upon knowledge changes and internalised risk assessments. All of these shifts of psychological drivers of behaviour must occur in a timely way and must work in harmony together. People must want to change their behaviour, must believe that the benefits of such behaviour change outweigh any costs, must feel good about making this change, must perceive that such behaviour change is expected by other people (especially those who represent important reference points or role models), and must believe they are capable of making this change. If a multitude of behaviour changes are required at the same time or within a fairly brief window of time, this can place a considerable psychological load on them (Aunger et al., 2016; Bashirian et al., 2020).

When Bish and Michie (2010) found that relatively few studies were theoretically grounded in the health sphere. When they were, there were two models that were utilised most often: the Health Belief Model and the Theory of Planned Behaviour. Other theories also surfaced in specific studies. Kupfer and colleagues studied the factors that motivated the practice of good hand hygiene using the Theory of Interpersonal Behaviour (Kupfer et al., 2019).

On examining research from earlier pandemics, Bish and Michie found many different psychological variables had been identified that could have shaped public behaviour. Sometimes, pandemic-related behaviour was influenced by risk perceptions which would include perceived risks to self and others and severity of disease once infected. Other studies examined whether people felt able to take protective steps and whether these steps were regarded as effective in the protection they could provide (King et al., 2016; Mitchell et al., 2009; Park et al., 2010; Rubin et al., 2009). Other variables of importance included demographic measures such as age, gender and ethnicity (Kamate et al., 2010; Kim, & Niederdeppe, 2013).

The Behaviour Change Wheel

The effectiveness of behavioural modelling as a scientific basis for policy during a pandemic requires that the right variables have been measured and that the selection of these variables is underpinned by an appropriate and tested theoretical framework. Critiquing this evidence, Michie and her colleagues concluded that other behavioural models often failed to deliver what was needed. Instead, a new system for configuring psychological theory to produce better quality research studies, which would inform public policy more effectively, was described and tested. Their review led this research group to identify 12 domains that could each play a part in contributing towards and explaining behaviour change (Michie et al., 2005).

This framework overlapped with but also went beyond the theory of planned behaviour. Important precursors to behaviour change, upon which behaviour change messages might work, were knowledge and skills, social and professional role and identity, beliefs about capabilities and about consequences, motivations and goals, memory, attention and decision making, environmental setting and resources, social influences, emotional regulation, behaviour regulation and nature of behaviour (Michie et al., 2005). Essentially, there were internal psychological processes linked to thoughts and beliefs, assessment of situations and problem-solving, assessment of ability to change behaviour, strength of intention to do so, and internal feelings about change. Then there were external factors linked to social and environmental conditions in which behaviour change was expected to take place.

The assessment of situations (which would include perceptions of risks and outcomes) is a familiar precursor to behaviour change for adherents to nudge theory. The alignment of beliefs and attitudes (or emotional feelings) and perceived ability to make change and control own behaviour in the ways expected, leading to intention to change behaviour are all components of the theory of planned behaviour model. The role also played by external factors is also credited equally to internal factors in the current model and this is given somewhat less attention in the other models.

In one practical example of how this might work, Michie and her colleagues referred to a campaign to promote the use of hand sanitiser in hospitals as an intervention designed to reduce the spread of infections. This behaviour might be especially important in emergency departments in which patients are seriously ill, undergo highly invasive treatment and may therefore be especially susceptible to infection. Yet, adoption of hand hygiene practices was slow in this setting. While the professionals that were present understood the significance of good hand hygiene, it was not used as often as expected.

Indeed, with the less urgent and serious procedures, hand hygiene was likely to be especially lax. Why? One explanation for this outcome was that it was linked to organisational resources and pressures. There were organisational constraints that encouraged rapid throughput of patients and these additional hygiene procedures were not always uppermost in the minds of the people who worked in these settings. Another possible factor was that some staffs were not always convinced that extra had sanitising made much difference to infection risks. The solution to this problem will derive from a more detailed understanding of the environmental setting and the priority perceptions of the people working there (Barrett & Cheung, 2021).

What this type of case study illustrates is that there may be no single solution to a real-world behaviour problem. How people will behave in different settings will be shaped by environmental factors as well as internal psychological assessments of situations by individuals. Many interventions in health and social policy contexts are presumed to be effective without empirical verification or theoretical reasoning behind them. Furthermore, when theory is considered, in the field of psychology and behaviour change, many different theoretical models have been developed that predict different outcomes. It might be useful to know whether more valuable lessons can be learned by amalgamating theories and combining their key strengths. In the presence of competing theories, however, it could be difficult to find a single behaviour-change prediction that is valid.

A range of theories might be used together in the hope that one hits the jackpot in terms of advising policy makers about the best ways to implement their policies to achieve desired public behaviour changes. This might still not solve the problem of choosing between theories. The efficacy of theories might be context-dependent. Moreover, some theories might have little value in one context but provide strong predictions in another. Another observation has been that certain parts of specific theories might prove to be effective at predicting specific behaviour change outcomes and not others. One way forward therefore would be to identify these theoretical predictors and eventually combine such elements from different theoretical models. In the past, disparate theories have sometimes produced common predictions of behaviour change outcomes in specific contexts, but their proponents were unable to explain how this agreement came about (Michie & Prestwich, 2010).

Williams (2010) commented on the article by Michie and Prestwich and while praising much of their work, pointed out that when trying to understand the impact of interventions on a target behaviour, the nature of the conditions in which comparisons were made needed to be articulated more thoroughly. In a subsequent response, Michie and her colleagues agreed that the more the efficacy of specific mechanisms that defined an intervention could be defined, the greater would be the confidence about the impact of different interventions (Michie et al., 2010).

Public information was important. It needed to be clear and to the point and communicate precisely the kinds of protective actions people could take. Where the public were being included as stakeholders who could play a central part in combating the spread of the virus, they needed to be told what they could do and how they could do it, and also the actions needed to be ones that people felt able to comply with. These principles were outlined by the COM-B model (capability-opportunity-motivation-behaviour (Michie & Perriard-Abdoh, 2020; Michie et al., 2014). This model formed part of a bigger framework of behaviour change, known as the Behaviour Change Wheel, which comprised 19 behaviour change formats (Michie, Van Stralen & West, 2011, 2014).

The Behaviour Change Wheel was devised as a new model for analysing the efficacy of social policies devised to produce public behaviour change. Many of the policies examined under this framework were linked to public health. Hence, the model was offered as a potentially useful framework for the analysis of behaviour change outcomes flowing from policies introduced during the COVID-19 pandemic. This behaviour analysis system considered three "conditions": capability, opportunity and motivation (the COM-B system). The wheel also comprised nine intervention functions that addressed deficits in one or more of these conditions. Then, there were seven types of policy in an outer rim that could create the conditions that would enable the interventions to occur.

Michie and her colleagues developed a model of behaviour change that began by identifying the different component parts of the behaviour change scenario under consideration before then identifying specific factors that might already underlie specific behaviour patterns and then interventions that might bring about the desired change (Michie, Abraham et al., 2011; Michie, Ashford et al. 2011). Within this approach an attempt was made to explore and itemise all types of intervention that had been shown empirically to have the potential to produce behaviour change. The initial scoping out work then identified the interventions known to provide the best fit for specific kinds of behaviour change in specific settings and when dealing with certain kinds of population.

This was regarded by its proponents as a more rigorous establishment process to ensure that any behaviour change campaign only utilised interventions about which there could be confidence underpinned by prior evidence. This approach meant that each behaviour change model was guided by science and not by what seemed to be logical or "common sense" intervention choices on the basis of the behaviour change challenge being confronted (Michie, Fixsen et al., 2009). Other popularly used behaviour changes, such as the theory of planned behaviour, failed to include specific factors that, according to past evidence, might also mediate the effectiveness of behaviour change campaigns, simply because they were never included as part of the original model (West, 2006).

Another observation here was the failure of previous behaviour change campaigns to choose between different theories to determine whether one model might be better than another as a framework for the behaviour change problem being addressed (Davies et al., 2010). Even worse, many campaigns were not driven by theory at all (Michie et al., 2005).

Finding a Fit between Macro-Level and Micro-Level Modelling

Another important modelling distinction to be made is between individual-level interventions and population-level interventions (National Institute for Health and Clinical Excellence, 2007). In the context of the SARS-CoV-2 pandemic, the epidemiology research that encouraged the British government to use a widespread "lockdown" of physical spaces in which people could intermingle, made its case based on macro-level (or population-level) modelling. This modelling originally concluded that if a number of key physical spaces and other broad categories of movement restrictions were deployed across the UK society, then the opportunities for the new virus to spread from person to person would be significantly reduced and this population-wide suite of interventions would bring the pandemic under control.

The "theory" here was perfectly sound. Eventually, it was found that it did work. What the original modelling did not and could not show, however, was how people, at the individual-level, would respond to such restrictions. The success of this strategy was ultimately dependent upon public behavioural compliance. Without it, the virus would continue to spread. Developing an effective persuasive campaign to encourage people to comply was a behavioural science problem.

What was also missing from the initial epidemiological modelling was any deconstruction of the unique effects of specific interventions even at a population-wide level. In addition, there was the associated problem of whether some interventions would prove to be less palatable than others to people in general or to specific sub-groups of the population but this was not a question for the mathematical modeller examining macro-level and non-pharmacological solutions to the accelerating spread of the new virus.

This type of scoping out of the behaviour change problem and whether specific component parts represent population-wide or individual-level issues then allows researchers to reflect on the analytical framework and methodology in more open-minded ways that are not constrained by the specific variables that customarily define a particular theory of behaviour change.

In effect, the Behaviour Wheel approach extracted solutions potentially from many different theoretical models. It might adopt other models in their entirety if all of their component parts were deemed to be relevant to the problem at hand, or otherwise specific component variables would be selected as deemed appropriate by the extant empirical evidence base and given the nature of the behaviour change problem.

In the context of the pandemic therefore when people were asked or required to suspend specific behaviours, many might have understood that there were good reasons for doing this but might nevertheless have found it difficult to comply if to do so meant that their lives were undermined to such an extent that the "cure" in this case caused more harm than the disease. It might be relevant, under such circumstances, to measure this type of perception because it could be expected to influence the degree of behavioural compliance people might be expected to exhibit. At the same time, it could be that a characteristic such as "impulsivity" was important as well because this determined, independently of subjective perceptions of being able to change one's behaviour, it made a difference to whether individuals would display tighter control over their own behaviour.

It is interesting to take note of the way the Behaviour Wheel approach evolved and the different types of variables that emerged as important component parts. Many of these were drawn from other theories of behaviour change (West et al., 2010). Following a systematic step-by-step protocol, Michie and her colleagues first identified key brain processes that motivated and directed behaviour. These included automatic and reflective factors. Next, three sets of behavioural measures were considered: the skills needed to perform a specific behaviour, an intention to do so, and the presence or absence of environmental constraints that might limit the target behaviour change. These three behavioural factors were summarised as capability, opportunity and motivation.

Individuals have got to have the physical and psychological abilities to perform specific behaviours. This means they must have all the necessary behavioural skills. There must be a sufficiently strong volition to perform that behaviour. Even though the individual might be able to stop smoking, do they really want to? If they are required to stay off work and remain at home, this could be a behaviour they could physically perform, but the economic circumstances of doing so would be too punitive, so they don't. This outcome might be reversed if the individual is encouraged to respond emotionally to the circumstances, for example, through fear that non-compliance might bring harm to themselves and to others close to them. There might also be a cognitive component through which appeals are made to beliefs that compliance would be civically responsible and also help ultimately to safeguard everybody.

What we can see here is a process of "working through" different permutations of variables that could be relevant to the achievement of the final, target behaviour. By applying this approach to the design of a behaviour change campaign, researchers are encouraged to consider a wide array of potentially effective interventions. They can then consult the research literature to find out whether there is compelling empirical evidence to substantiate the behaviour change efficacy of specific interventions. Models such as nudge theory, group processes/social identity theory and the theory of planned behaviour comprise pre-defined packages of precursors to behaviour change that did not attempt to look further at other potential determinants of behaviour change. When considering the opportunity to change behaviour, context becomes all important. Behaviour change might be internally motivated to occur, but whether it is followed through to completion depends upon whether the environment puts up physical or psychological barriers in the way.

Through this more open-ended analysis of factors that could, theoretically, play a part in changing behaviour, those eventually selected to guide the implementation of specific interventions depended not only on whether they had ever been shown to be effective but also on whether they were likely to be effective in the specific context being considered. Some interventions might work very well to encourage people to change their eating habits, but would then have little impact on encouraging compliance with pandemic lockdown restrictions. In developing a theoretical or analytical model for a specific setting therefore it is essential to be confident that chosen interventions are likely to work in the specific setting in which they are being used.

The Behaviour Change Wheel purports to provide a method for mapping out the interventions that might be most effective in the specific behavioural setting being examined. Target behaviours might be well within the capabilities of most people and many could have the internal motivation to perform them, but within the setting being considered the willing adoption of those behaviours might not be straightforward for everybody.

Behavioural Modelling and Early Pandemic Policy

It was suggested by some observers, that the British government initially adopted a policy of "herd immunity" rather than societal lockdown. One rationale for this, it was claimed, was a concern that public behavioural compliance would run out of steam quite quickly – a so-called compliance fatigue effect. No evidence was offered for this view. No theoretical rationale was presented to substantiate the possibility it might occur. Others denied that this had ever been a government policy. Nonetheless, the decision of whether to lock down or not to lockdown was taken, encouraged by macro-level epidemiological modelling.

What was not known at the outset, however, was whether all the recommended lockdown interventions were necessary and which ones were likely to have the greatest individual impact. It was not known either whether some of these behavioural restrictions would be found more difficult to sustain over time than others at the individual level. These are important questions. The answers to them could provide insights into the order in which to relax lockdown restrictions and whether it would be necessary in a future crisis of this sort, including second or third waves of COVID-19, to shut all the physical spaces that were compulsorily closed in the first lockdown (Michie, Abraham et al., 2011; Michie, Ashford et al. 2011; Michie, Fixsen et al., 2009).

Following on from the points being made earlier about context and selection of interventions that make the best fit for behaviour change, Michie and her colleagues identified "domain-specific" behaviour change interventions. These were developed for behaviour change in relation to alcohol consumption, tobacco smoking and physical activity (Michie & Johnston, 2012; Michie et al., 2015). This research reviewed past scientific evidence and used depth interviews with a sample of over 40 international experts. Nearly 100 different behaviour change techniques were identified that were further grouped into 16 categories. This provided a reference source for devising more context-specific and targeted models of behaviour change analysis. As the SARS-CoV-2 pandemic took hold in the United Kingdom, the researchers behind the Behaviour Change Wheel called for research to be carried out on probable public compliance with each of the many behavioural restrictions imposed during the first British lockdown (West et al., 2020). Behaviour restrictions would be crucial set of tools to use in bringing the pandemic under control. Many physical spaces had been closed anyway and this meant that people could not meet with each other there. Other important behaviours, such as not meeting people from other households in your own home, wearing face masks in those indoor spaces that remained open, regular handwashing and diligently socially isolating when symptomatic were dependent on people's voluntary compliance (Michie, 2020).

The implementation of non-pharmaceutical interventions (NPIs) such as physical distancing could only be effective if there was full public compliance with them. This meant that the authorities, that is, governments and their public health systems, depended upon the members of the public taking a degree of personal responsibility for their own well-being and the protection of others. This mindset was endorsed by the World Health Organization whose director-general called upon,

> Every individual [to] understand that they are not helpless – there are things everyone should do to protect themselves and others. Your

health is in your hands. That includes physical distancing, hand hygiene, covering coughs, staying home if you fell sick, wearing masks when appropriate, and only sharing information from reliable sources. (British Psychological Society, 2020)

Getting people to change their behaviours to this extent, however, needed external support. This meant that the right conditions needed to be created for individuals and also for entire communities that would encourage widespread compliance (Michie, West, Amlot & Rubin, 2020). No single measure or set of measures were likely to be effective on their own. A multifaceted approach was needed to ensure an NPI-based system of pandemic control would work (van Bavel et al., 2020). In any health campaign that targets a specific type of behaviour change on a population-wide basis, a firm scientific understanding of the efficacy of interventions was needed. In terms of whether people do change their behaviour, it is always important to understand their perceptions of the significance of this change, their willingness and ability to change, and their responsiveness to encouragements or discouragements to do so that emanated from the environment around them (Shah, 2020; Taylor, 2019).

Epidemiological models recommended that governments should deploy a wide range of physical distancing and other measures to slow the spread of SARS-CoV-2. The recommended interventions were usually presented to governments in "blocks" or "groupings" of restrictions. Models predicted viral spread outcomes with and without these block interventions. What was made less clear was the relative contribution to the outcome of a slower spreading disease of specific interventions, such as closures of bars, cafes and restaurants, closures of leisure and entertainment venues, school closures, shop closures, and so on (Michie, Abraham et al., 2009).

Yet, behavioural scientists, in the past, found that behaviour change interventions could have varying effects on the ways people behaved in relation to their health (Bootsma & Ferguson, 2007; Hatchett, Mecher & Lipsitch, 2007; Mitchell et al., 2009). Certain combinations of techniques proved to be more effective than others. To inform lessons from the SARS-CoV-2 pandemic, to guide decisions about sequencing of intervention release, and to guide the development of effective interventions models in the future, research that disentangled the effects of different intervention variables and combinations of such variables on specified measured outcomes was identified as a priority (Cane et al., 2015).

As earlier chapters showed, it is possible to get people to adopt new behaviours and suspend existing actions through a range of influences, some of which address internal psychological changes to attitudes, beliefs and behavioural intentions, some of which make reference to surrounding social settings and groups, and some of which utilise environmental cues. Each of these approaches, as we will see, can produce beneficial results.

Often, though, they need to be combined if powerful and sustainable behaviour change is needed in a hurry. Moving forward, the book now turns to the application of the four behaviour change models in relation to public compliance with physical distancing restrictions and adoption of protective behaviours.

References

Aunger, R., Greenland, K., Ploubidis, G., Schmidt, W., Oxford, J., & Curtis, V. (2016). The determinants of reported personal and household hygiene behaviour: A multi-country study. *PLoS One, 11*(8), e0159551.

Barrett, C., & Cheung, K. L. (2021). Knowledge, socio-cognitive perceptions and the practice of hand hygiene and social distancing during the COVID-19 pandemic: A cross-sectional study of UK university students. *BMC Public Health, 21,* Article 426.

Bashirian, S., Jenabi, E., Khazaei, S., Karimi-Shahanjarini, A., Zareian, S., et al. (2020). Factors associated with preventive behaviours of COVID-19 among hospital staff in Iran in 2020: An application of the protection motivation theory. *Journal of Hospital Infections, 105*(3), 430–433.

Bavel, J. J. V., Baicker, K., Boggio, P. S., Capraro, V., Cichocka, A., Cikara, M., Crockett, M. J., Crum, A. J., Douglas, K. M., Druckman, J. N., Drury, J., Dube, O., Ellemers, N., Finkel, E. J., Fowler, J. H., Gelfand, M., Han, S., Haslam, S. A., Jetten, J., Kitayama, S., ... (2020). Using social and behavioural science to support COVID-19 pandemic response. *Nature and Human Behaviour, 4*(5), 460–471. https://doi.org/10.1038/s41562-020-0884-z

Bish, A., & Michie, S. (2010). Demographic and attitudinal determinants of protective behaviours during a pandemic: A review. *British Journal of Health Psychology, 15*(4), 797–824.

Bootsma, M. C., & Ferguson, N. M. (2007). The effect of public health measures on the 1918 influenza pandemic in U.S. cities. *Proceedings of the National Academy of Science USA, 104*(18), 7588–7593. https://doi.org/10.1073/pnas.0611071104

British Psychological Society. (2020). Behavioural science and disease prevention taskforce. *Behavioural Science and Disease Prevention: Psychological Guidance.* https://www.bps.org.uk/sites/www.bps.org.uk/files/Policy/Policy %20-%20Files/Behavioural%20science%20and%20disease%20prevention %20-%20Psychological%20guidance%20for%20optimising%20policies%20 and%20communication.pdf

Cane, J., Richardson, M., Johnston, M., Ladha, R., & Michie, S. (2015). From lists of behaviour change techniques (BCTs) to structured hierarchies: Comparison of two methods of developing a hierarchy of BCTs. *British Journal of Health Psychology, 20*(1), 130–150. https://doi.org/10.1111/bjhp.12102. Epub 12 May 2014.

Davies, P., Walker, A. E., & Grimshaw, J. M. (2010). A systematic review of the use of theory in the design of guideline dissemination and implementation strategies and interpretation of the results of rigorous evaluations. *Implementation Science, 5,* 14.

Hatchett, R. J., Mecher, C. E., & Lipsitch, M. (2007). Public health interventions and epidemic intensity during the 1918 influenza pandemic. *Proceedings of the National Academy of Science U S A., 104*(18), 7582–7587. https://doi.org/10.1 073/pnas.0610941104

Institute for Government. (2010). *MINDSPACE: Influencing Behaviour through Public Policy.* London, UK: Institute for Government, the Cabinet Office.

Kamate, S. K., Agrawal, A., Chaudhary, H., Singh, K., Mishra, P., & Asawa, K. (2010). Public knowledge, attitude and behavioural changes in an Indian population during the influenza A (H1N1) outbreak. *Journal of Infection in Developing Countrie, 4*(1), 7.

Kim, H. K., & Niederdeppe, J. (2013). Exploring optimistic bias and the integrative model of behavioral prediction in the context of a campus influenza outbreak. *Journal of Health Communication, 18*(2), 206–222.

King, D. B., Kamble, S., & DeLongis, A. (2016). Coping with influenza A/H1N1 in India: empathy is associated with increased vaccination and health precautions. *International Journal of Health Promotion and Education, 54*(6), 283–294.

Kupfer, T. R., Wyles, K. J., Watson, F., La Ragione, R. M., Chambers, M. A., & Macdonald, A. S. (2019). Determinants of hand hygiene behaviour based on the theory of interpersonal behaviour. *Journal of Infection Prevention, 20*(5), 232–237.

Mansdorf, I. J. (2020, 18th March). Enforcing compliance with COVID-19 pandemic restrictions: Psychological aspects of a national security threat. *PreventionWeb.* Retrieved from: https://www.preventionweb.net/news/view/ 70917

Michie, S. (2020). Behavioural, environmental, social and systems interventions against covid-19. *thebmj, 370.* https://doi.org/10.1136/bmj.m2982

Michie, S., Abraham, C., Eccles, M. P., Francis, J. J., Hardeman, W., & Johnston, M. (2011). Strengthening evaluation and implementation by specifying components of behaviour change interventions: A study protocol. *Implementation Science, 7*(6), 10. https://doi.org/10.1186/1748-5908-6-10

Michie, S., Abraham, C., Eccles, M. P., Francis, J. J., Hardeman, W., & Johnston, M. (2011). Strengthening evaluation and implementation by specifying components of behaviour change interventions: A study protocol. *Implementation Science, 6,* 10. https://doi.org/10.1186/1748-5908-6-10

Michie, S., Abraham, C., Whittington, C., McAteer, J., & Gupta, S. (2009). Effective techniques in healthy eating and physical activity interventions: A meta-regression. *Health Psychology, 28*(6), 690–701.

Michie, S., Ashford, S., Sniehotta, F. F., Dombrowski, S. U., Bishop, A., & French, D. P. (2011). A refined taxonomy of behaviour change techniques to help people change their physical activity and healthy eating behaviours: The CALO-RE taxonomy. *Psychology and Health, 26*(11), 1479–1498. https://doi.org/10.1080/ 08870446.2010.540664

Michie, S., Atkins, L., & West, R. (2014). *The Behaviour Change Wheel: A Guide to Designing Interventions.* London, UK: Silverback Publishing.

Michie, S., Fixsen, D., Grimshaw, J. M., & Eccles, M. P. (2009). Specifying and reporting complex behaviour change interventions: The need for a scientific method. *Implementation Science*, *4*, Article number 40. Retrieved from: https://implementationscience.biomedcentral.com/articles/10.1186/1748-5908-4-40

Michie, S., & Johnston, M. (2012). Theories and techniques of behaviour change: Developing a cumulative science of behaviour change. *Health Psychology Review*, *6*, 1–6.

Michie, S., Johnston, M., Abraham, C., Lawton, R., Parker, D., & Walker, A. (2005). "Psychological Theory" group. Making psychological theory useful for implementing evidence-based practice: A consensus approach. *Quality and Safety in Health Care*, *14*(1), 26–33. https://doi.org/10.1136/qshc.2004.011155

Michie, S., & Perriard-Abdoh, S. (2020, 27th March). Informing and translating the evidence base. *The Psychologist*. Retrieved from: https://thepsychologist.bps.org.uk/informing-and-translating-evidence-base

Michie, S., & Prestwich, A. (2010). Are interventions theory-based? Development of a theory coding scheme. *Health Psychology*, *29*(1), 1–8. https://doi.org/10.1037/a0016939

Michie, S., Prestwich, A., & de Bruin, M. (2010). Importance of the nature of comparison conditions for testing theory-based interventions: Reply. *Health Psychology*, *29*(5), 468–470. https://doi.org/10.1037/a0020844

Michie, S., Van Stralen, M. M., & West, R. (2011). The behaviour change wheel: A new method for characterising and designing behaviour change interventions. *Implementation Science*, *6*(1), Article number 42. Retrieved from: https://implementationscience.biomedcentral.com/articles/10.1186/1748-5908-6-42

Michie, S., West, R., Amiot, R., & Rubin, J. (2020). Slowing down the covid-19 outbreak: changing behaviour by understanding it. *BMJ Opinion*. https://blogs.bmj.com/bmj/2020/03/11/slowing-down-the-covid-19-outbreak-changing-behaviour-by-understanding-it/

Michie, S., Wood, C. E., Johnston, M., Abraham, C., Francis, J. J., & Hardeman, W. (2015). Behaviour change techniques: The development and evaluation of a taxonomic method for reporting and describing behaviour change interventions (a suite of five studies involving consensus methods, randomised controlled trials and analysis of qualitative data). *Health Technology Assessment*, *19*(99), 1–188. https://doi.org/10.3310/hta19990 (Top of form).

Mitchell, T., Dee, D. L., Phares, C. R., Lipman, H. B., Gould, L. H., Kutty, P., et al. (2009). Non-pharmaceutical interventions during an outbreak of 2009 pandemic influenza A (H1N1) virus infection at a large public university. Clinical and Infectious Disorders, *52*(Suppl. 1), S138–S145.

National Institute for Health and Clinical Excellence. (2007). *Behaviour Change at Population, Community and Individual Levels (Public Health Guidance 6)*. London: NICE.

Park, J. H., Cheong, H. K., Son, D. Y., Kim, S. U., & Ha, C. M. (2010). Perceptions and behaviors related to hand hygiene for the prevention of H1N1 influenza transmission among Korean university students during the peak pandemic period. *BMC Infectious Diseases*, *10*(1), 222.

Rubin, G. J., Amlôt, R., Page, L., & Wessely, S. (2009). Public perceptions, anxiety, and behaviour change in relation to the swine flu outbreak: Cross sectional telephone survey. *BMJ*, *339*(7713), 156.

Shah, H. (2020). Global problems need social science. *Nature, 577*(7790), 295. Retrieved from: https://www.nature.com/articles/d41586-020-00064-x

Taylor, S. (2019). *The Psychology of Pandemics: Preparing for the Next Global Outbreak of Infectious Disease.* Newcastle, UK: Cambridge Scholars Publishing.

West, R. (2006). *Theory of Addiction.* Oxford, UK: Blackwells.

West, R., Michie, S., Rubin, G. J. et al. (2020). Applying principles of behaviour change to reduce SARS-CoV-2 transmission. *Natural Human Behaviour, 4,* 451–459. https://doi.org/10.1038/s41562-020-0887-9

West, R., Walia, A., Hyder, N., Shahab, L., & Michie, S. (2010). Behavior change techniques used by the English Stop Smoking Services and their associations with short-term quit outcomes. *Nicotine Tobacco Research, 12*(7), 742–747.

Williams, D. M. (2010). Importance of the nature of comparison conditions for testing theory-based interventions: Comment on Michie and Prestwich (2010). *Health Psychology, 29*(5), 467. https://doi.org/10.1037/a0019597

Chapter 6

Nudge Theory and Physical Distancing

Nudge techniques are based on inserting subtle signals to people about how to behave in specific environments and settings. These may take the form of messages piped through the mainstream media or over the online world or signs and cues within physical environments. One often-cited example of nudging behaviour in the real world is a technique that was used in men's urinals to encourage them not to miss the target. Overflows caused by men not paying attention to where they are urinating incurs additional clean-up costs in men's public conveniences. One city painted an image of a fly on their urinals that invited men to use it as a target. The result was that fewer men missed the target and less collateral mess occurred as a result (Klein, 2020).

As noted earlier in this book, the Nobel Prize winning psychologists, Amos Tversky and Daniel Kahneman, inspired the nudge approach through their experimental cognitive psychological experiments on risk judgements and environmental cues. Personal assessments of event frequencies were found to be based less on their objective likelihood of occurrence and more on subjective calculations of their probability that were influenced by recent or highly salient experiences of these events. A rare event would be subjectively evaluated as more frequently occurring than it really was if an individual had had a recent direct or indirect experience of it. That experience would bring that event to the "top of mind" and cause an individual to believe that it was more frequently occurring simply because they had a relatively recent experience of it (Tversky & Kahneman, 1973, 1979).

Nudge theory was more recently popularised by the writings of Cass Sunstein (a legal theorist) and Richard Thaler (a behavioural economist). It was their work that encouraged a number of national governments, including the United Kingdom, to adopt its techniques to understand better how to change public behaviour to comply with new public policies (Thaler & Sunstein, 2008). The behaviour-change techniques adopted by this perspective were often subtle and relatively non-invasive. They used cues and prompts inserted into environments in which behaviour change was sought. These signals to people as to how to behave in specific settings could also be reinforced with messaging that informed people about behaviour outcomes,

DOI: 10.4324/9781003274308-6

with a focus on manipulating people's risk assessments associated with different behavioural choices.

Scientists, familiar with previous pandemics and how to tackle them, knew from the start that it might be necessary to deploy more invasive measures that would place severe constraints on public behaviour. At the outset of this new pandemic, however, there was probably a general and somewhat optimistic hope that such measures would not prove to be necessary and that other "softer" approaches could be deployed that would slow the spread of the virus. This was important not exclusively because the politicians and experts were concerned about the public, but because their main concern was that if large numbers of people were made seriously ill by this new virus, and needed special care and treatment, hospitals could be overwhelmed.

Nudge approaches have been commonly used in many behaviour-change contexts and people often respond well to them (Sunstein, 2016; Sunstein et al., 2018). Nudges represent one of the softer approaches to public behaviour change and for that reason have been accepted by the public (Diepeveen et al., 2013; Hagmann et al., 2018). Having said that, as we will see, there are "hard" and "soft" forms of nudging and in the former case, more direct instructions might be issued by authorities about how people should change their behaviour in specific settings.

The tension between effectiveness and popularity of government-imposed restrictions on public behaviour has created a climate for more research to help everyone understand how to use nudge approaches optimally (Sunstein et al., 2019). Part of this effort has focused on learning more about how different kinds of people react to specific types of restrictions (Jung & Mellers, 2016). This work has found that these restrictions might be received better by people in particular demographic groups, or who are characterised by specific personality attributes or simply on the basis of perceptions of fairness and justification of these interventions (Reynolds et al., 2018).

Within the context of the COVID-19 pandemic, governments were confronted with a crisis for which medical or pharmaceutical protections were not initially available. The new disease was spreading very quickly such as hospitals were put under a lot of strain and new policies were needed – and fast – to bring disease transmission under control. Much initial focus was placed on personal hygiene measures and some initial measures emphasised control of surface transmission as much as airborne transmission. Once it was established that the disease was mostly airborne, government policies had to change. Nudging people into making behaviour changes became the order of the day.

Application of Nudge Theory during the Pandemic

Around the world, national governments varied in their initial responses to the pandemic. After initial cases of COVID-19 had been recorded, some governments quickly closed down their societies. Others carried on largely as normal with a few warnings to their populations about taking greater care in specific settings. In the case of this pandemic, the British government at first advised people to wash their hands more and for those operating physical spaces (e.g., offices, retail outlets, leisure and sports venues and others) to clean down surfaces that people had touched. Some additional advisories were posted about avoidance of some physical spaces where large numbers of people might gather in close proximity to each other. It stopped short of closing down such events. For example, just a short time before there was a radical change of strategy, the Cheltenham Festival was allowed to happen with thousands in attendance at a big horse race meeting (Davidson, 2020; Wood & Carroll, 2020). News surfaced that some racegoers subsequently displayed COVID-19 symptoms which they were believed to have acquired at this event (Mortimer, 2020).

COVID-19 Experiences, Risk Awareness and Fear

Risk perceptions can be fuelled by a variety of factors. Objective assessments of risk can be made from data about infection rates and death rates, especially among specific social groups. This input can strike home if the individual happens to fall demographically within population sub-groups most widely infected and therefore most "at risk". Even when "objective" or mathematically calculated risks are quite low, a perceived risk (or "subjective" risk) can emerge that exaggerates the actual risk from an individual's personal perspective.

Subjective risks are not invariably calculated by people through rational analysis of relevant evidence. Such risks can be shaped and magnified by someone's personal experiences; by the personal evidence supplied by others with whom an individual interacts, knows well, and trusts; by information provided through the mass media (especially from trusted media sources); and more generally by their life experiences and emergent view of the world. These experiences can render even statistically rare occurrences to be apparently more frequently occurring than they really are. One major investigation provided evidence early on about initial public risk perceptions linked to COVID-19 and the factors that played a part in shaping them.

Sarah Dryhurst and her colleagues at the University of Cambridge investigated COVID-19 risk perceptions in different parts of the world. They obtained their data from 6,991 respondents spread across ten countries. They found that levels of concern were quite high everywhere, but highest of all in the United Kingdom. A range of predictors of concern and risk were identified. These included personal experience with the virus, interactions with family and friends, trust in government, medical professionals and other scientists, knowledge of government strategy, perceived efficacy in dealing with the virus and other personal factors (Dryhurst et al., 2020).

Risk was measured by Dryhurst and her colleagues in terms of perceived likelihood on the part of respondents that they or members of their family would contract the coronavirus in the next six months and their level of worry about this. On a seven-point risk-perception index, average coronavirus risk scores across the sampled countries varied between 4.78 and 5.45. This level of variance produced some statistically significant differences between pairs of countries.

In determining factors that might have contributed to this risk perception, the researchers ran regression analyses to discover which variables among those on which they collected data from respondents emerged as the best predictors of perceived risk. They found that personal experience with the virus, information received from family and friends, their tendency towards "prosociality", an individualistic view of the world and perceptions that they personally and the world more generally could cope with this new virus were among the strongest predictors. There was also a general tendency for women to perceive greater risk on average than did men (Dryhurst et al., 2020).

Having had direct personal experience with the virus, triggered greater perceived risk associated with it. Those individuals that had received a lot of information and comment from family and friends also held stronger perceptions of risk from COVID-19. Those individuals that believe it is important to do things for others, even when there may be personal costs from doing so, perceived greater risk. Having an individualistic view of the world, whereby catering to your personal ambitions and success outweigh in importance of working towards the betterment of your social group or community (a collectivistic worldview) predicted weaker perceived risk from the coronavirus. When individuals thought they could take steps personally to protect themselves from this virus, they perceived more risk from it. However, those who judged their community or country to be able collectively to deal with this virus effectively also regarded the risks from it as reduced. Having greater trust in science, in medical practitioners and in government resulted in lower risk perceptions. Having greater personal knowledge about the virus was also a source of comfort and weakened risk perceptions.

There were variances in how significant these different predictor variables turned out to be in different countries. While these predictor variables were linked significantly to risk perceptions for the world sample, they did not always emerge as significant in specific countries. Holding individualistic worldviews, for example, was a significant predictor of risk perception in the United Kingdom, Germany, Sweden, Spain and Japan, but not in other countries. Overall, individualism accounted for 4.78% of the variance in risk perceptions around the world and was the strongest predictor variable of them all. Prosociality, that is, caring about others before yourself, was the second strongest predictor (3.19% of variance in risk perception) but did not emerge as significant in every country. It was especially weak as a predictor of risk perception in South Korea (Dryhurst et al., 2020).

Direct experience with the virus (2.34% of variance) was another important predictor and was especially strong in the United States and South Korea, but was weak in Australia. Trust in medical practitioners (1.73%) and in science (1.62%) emerged among the strongest predictors of risk perceptions overall and especially in South Korea. Personal efficacy (1.62% overall) was important as a predictor of risk perception in Germany and Sweden, but less so elsewhere (Dryhurst et al., 2020). There was some evidence also that taking preventative health measures such as washing hands, wearing face masks and adhering to physical distancing were linked to risk perceptions and tended to reduce feelings of being at risk. Risk perceptions can be important motivators of these behaviours on the part of individuals during pandemics (Bish & Michie, 2010; Rudisill, 2013; Wise et al., 2020).

What did emerge from this research was that having had close contact with the virus through direct experience or the experience of others close to you can significantly impact your own perceptions of risk from it. Sources close to you have potentially the greatest impact of this sort (Slovic et al., 2004; van der Linden, 2014, 2015; Weber, 2006). It is possible that a more direct experience of this kind creates a more concrete and explicit mindset about the virus and its effects (Trope & Liberman, 2010). Finally, though, the predictor variables used in the Dryhurst study accounted for just 26% of the variance in coronavirus risk perceptions. This meant that nearly three-quarters of the variance in these perceptions remained unexplained. There is therefore still plenty of additional research needed to discover other factors that shape these perceptions and which therefore might nudge people towards certain behaviour, following on from their risk assessments. Even so, we can conclude, that direct and indirect experiences from an individual's own life can exert a significant impact on public awareness and concern about a pandemic. Such concerns are then likely to motivate people, at least for a time, to alter their usual behaviour patterns.

Associations between Nudging and Social Distancing

Researchers in the United States investigated public compliance with social distancing measures during the first wave of SARS-CoV-2 during March, April and May 2020 in five states that had accounted for half of all COVID-19 cases in the country. Data were gathered in case numbers, public mobility patterns, and the rate of infection transmission in California, Illinois, Massachusetts, New Jersey and New York (Liu et al., 2021).

These five states had all mandated social distancing rules during the same period (19th–24th March). There was evidence that public compliance with these restrictions already showed signs of waning by mid-April. Across the period being studied, the daily reproduction number decreased from a high of over two to over five in the different states to under or just over one. At the start of this period, social distancing compliance was high but decreased over time in all five states. There was evidence that people gradually started to move around more and visited more locations where they encountered others. There was some evidence, nonetheless, that areas where public compliance with social distancing was greater also had lower infection rates and brought the rate of infection under control better.

A further US study of social distancing measures framed within a nudge approach confirmed that these interventions could bring health benefits to populations during a pandemic crisis. This study collected data from the same participants over time (Siedner et al., 2020). In a field experiment, they tested the impact of the introduction of social distancing measures and internal movement restrictions on COVID-19 infection transmission rates. Initial data collection, at different data points occurred up to 14 days before social distancing measures to three days afterwards and the second data collection point was between four and 14 days after these interventions had been implemented.

The researchers measured state-wide COVID-19 case growth rate and also mortality rate from this virus. No evidence emerged of significant internal movement restriction effects on infection rates, but it was difficult to disentangle the impact of this intervention from parallel social distancing interventions. If social distancing did have an impact, it was not felt initially. In fact, COVID-19 attributed death rates increased for a small amount over the first seven days after social distancing was introduced. Afterwards, however, there was evidence that social distancing effects did kick in after a further seven days and that infection levels dropped. This apparent effect of social distancing weakened beyond seven days. Moreover, changes in infection and death rates could also have been linked to changes in other factors such as increased numbers of COVID tests being completed that meant greater detection of cases over time because of better detection and reporting.

Dutch research also examined nudging and social distancing effects. The researchers observed that public compliance with such restrictions was essential to their eventual success. It was important therefore not simply to catalogue that social distancing rules had been implemented but also to establish as confidently as possible that the public actually went along with these restrictions. One of the weaknesses of a lot of research on lockdown effects is that there is a reliance on what people tell researchers, but when it comes to their actual behaviour very little validation of these reports is provided. In this investigation, the researchers used closed-circuit television footage of public behaviour in inner-city Amsterdam to find out if people were observing the 1.5 metre social distancing rule when walking around in public settings (Hoeben et al., 2021).

The findings showed that people seemed mostly to comply with these rules when they were initially introduced. Thereafter, public compliance gradually waned. The more crowded streets became, the more often there were breaches of the social distancing rules. Further data from cell phones showed that quite a few people were tracked as having left their homes, despite a well-publicised stay at home rule. Further analysis indicated that greater non-compliance with these rules did exhibit a statistical relationship to changes in transmission rates of COVID-19. The latter variable was also related to the numbers of COVID-related Google searches performed during this period and media attention to COVID-19.

What this study showed was even though opinion polls might report that large proportions of national populations might accept and follow restrictions on their behaviour, more direct, observational or live movement tracking data revealed that their claims may not be borne out by their behaviour. Such evidence indicates that if nudging methods are to be used to control public behaviour, live behaviour monitoring could provide valuable planning insights into the public spaces where people are most likely to be non-compliant. These are the locations where localised nudge cues and signals that provide on the spot influences should be most often deployed.

A Korean study investigated nudging techniques during the COVID-19 pandemic and made comparisons with the 2015 Middle East Respiratory Syndrome coronavirus outbreak (Jang et al., 2020). Data were obtained for 2nd and 25th June 2015 and between 4th February and 2nd April 2020. More than 4,000 participants were interviewed. Data were collected about compliance with social distancing measures and adoption of self-protective behaviours such as handwashing and wearing face masks. There was more widespread social distancing practised during the 2020 pandemic (83–92%) than in the 2015 pandemic (42–58%) across surveys conducted at different time points in each pandemic. The Korean public was also far more likely to adopt self-protective measures during COVID-19 (79–80%) than during the MERS outbreak (16% up to a high of 60%). During both pandemics, people who perceived the greatest amount of risk were more likely to comply with these behaviours.

Optimistic Bias and COVID-19 Perceptions and Behaviour

People did vary in their reactions to these messages from government. It was noted previously that people vary in their degree of optimism when it comes to personal risks. There is a tendency often for people to believe that bad outcomes are more likely to be experienced by other people than by themselves (Harris et al., 2008; Hoorens, 2008; Weinstein, 1980). This might have led some people to flout the rules and break lockdown guidelines in the belief that the risks from which they were advised to protect themselves did not really apply to them (Curtis, 2020; Duffy, 2020).

Some rule-breaking might also be explained by a failure to understand the rules and restrictions rather than by deliberate defiance. Other people may have found that the collateral effects of lockdown were so bad that they would rather take their chances with COVID-19 (Duffy, 2020). Some people were undoubtedly extremely bored by their social isolation and other experienced symptoms of loneliness. There was also evidence from the past that the more optimistic in the population were also inclined to take more risks anyway. It might be expected therefore that these individuals would take chances (Burger & Burns, 1988; Radcliffe & Klein, 2002).

One of the issues confronted by behavioural scientists seeking to use behaviour change and control as a tool to tackle a pandemic is how to balance people's perceptions of risks against their self-confidence that they can cope by managing the risk. Sometimes, people are known to over-estimate their own security against risk as compared with others. Some people might believe their own chances of infection are lower than that of others. They might also believe that if they do get infected, they will get less seriously ill than most other people. This psychological phenomenon is known as "optimistic bias" in nudge literature.

Researchers at Kings College London discovered that many of their study's participants felt less at risk from COVID-19 than other people. This did not they actually were at less risk but merely that this is what they believed. Optimistic bias had been witnessed in many other settings (Kings College London, 2020). Optimism leads some people to believe that they are less likely than others to experience negative events and more likely to experience positive ones. The worry here is that such beliefs might lead these individuals to take unnecessary risks when confronted with potentially hazardous situations.

More optimistic people were also known to be less anxious and hence in the context of the pandemic, they were probably more inclined to challenge restrictive rules concerning their own behaviour because they were less easily frightened into submission (Ruthig et al., 2007). Relative optimism therefore was a double-edged sword and while it might render some people as more likely to take risks, when the world opened up again, they were more likely to put themselves at risk in embracing restored freedoms of movement (Taylor & Brown, 1988, 1994).

One survey of social media users in the United Kingdom between the fifth and eighth weeks of the first lockdown found that people could be differentiated in terms of their optimism bias. Some expressed greater optimism when they also believed they were less likely than others to be infected by the novel coronavirus or to need hospitalisation or intensive care if they did become infected. This initial optimism did not mean that they never felt at risk, however. Some of these individuals were still aware that they could be at risk of infection in the future (Asimakopoulou et al., 2020).

These findings of optimism bias could vary across demographics. This judgement varied among women and men and among different age groups. Much depended on the perceived controllability of specific events. When individuals were asked about events over which they felt they had some control, their optimism would surface. With events that they believed were not so controllable, this self-confidence would evaporate. Those with optimism therefore did not dismiss the possibility that they would become infected, but they were more confident than others that they would not be made seriously ill. If they did get ill, they were also more confident about making a full recovery.

Unlike earlier research, this survey found that there was pessimism about the future. Previously, evidence has shown that optimistic bias can grow stronger when people are making judgements about events that are some distance off in the future (Carroll et al., 2006; Shepperd et al., 2000). This finding was not replicated here. There was evidence from this survey, consistent with past research, that those with ill health were more pessimistic than most others about their chances of experiencing poor health in the future (Asimakopoulou et al., 2008).

In the context of the pandemic, initial requests from government, which eventually were issued like instructions, focused on telling people to stay home and avoid close physical contact with others with whom they did not already live. This could be seen as a controllable request with which many could and would readily comply – in the short term. As a longer-term option, however, this would have been seen by many as an option that could pose serious compliance problems for them. No amount of nudging was likely to change this.

As we will see in chapter Eight, when behaviour change or control requests are perceived as non-feasible or simply beyond their capability to obey, it may be less likely to occur. The theory of planned behaviour is built out of constructs that represent this idea and research conducted under this theoretical framework, including about public responses to the pandemic, has shown that this construct of "perceived behaviour control" is critical to the conditioning of behaviour change and compliance. Knowing this, it follows that the imposition of interventions such as social isolation should only ever be envisaged as short-term options. They might prove very effective in bringing rampant spread of a new virus under control, especially when its transmission is mostly through the air, following the outbreak of a new disease. It needs to be applied sufficiently comprehensively to have a real impact. This means it must command widespread compliance across a population. Yet, it must be recognised that such compliance will probably have a short shelf life. When optimism that a course of action is working turns to pessimism, keeping public behaviour in check, could prove to be more problematic (Chambers et al., 2003).

Loss Aversion and Public Behaviour during the Pandemic

The concept of loss aversion was introduced by Tversky and Kahneman (1979). When people make judgements, they found, they tend to attach more weight to potential losses they can envisage than to potential benefits that might be accrued. The size of the losses and the size of the gains might be more or less the same in their actual weight of impact, but this is not usually the way they are perceived. One outcome of this phenomenon is that people may be more willing to take bigger risks to avoid losses than to gain benefits (Haigh & List, 2005). These judgements have been found to work across a range of settings including in the context of health-related decision making (Farrell et al., 2006). This evidence was thought to have important implications for the way the risks associated with COVID-19 were framed in order to achieve specific behaviour control outcomes. More nudging success might be forthcoming in getting people to comply with behaviour restrictions if doing so was framed in terms of losses avoided rather than benefits gain (Bavel et al., 2020).

As an example of health influences, research had found that it was effective to some degree in relation to changing smoking habits. Ultimately, however, the effectiveness of specific nudging frames is related to the relative certainty (or uncertainty) about the outcome (Rothman & Salovey, 1997). In the case of the COVID-19 pandemic, there were so many uncertainties because of the limited understanding of the new coronavirus that existed at the time of its initial outbreak. With greater uncertainty, loss frames have been found to become more appealing and persuasive (Rothman & Salovey, 1997).

Researchers at Kings College London with experience in nudge research used this methodology to study the public's behavioural reactions to the COVID-19 pandemic. Despite previous findings showing that subtle psychological cues could be effective in shaping people's behaviour patterns in different settings, these responses were not always replicated in the same way for COVID-19.

In fact, the Kings College researchers questioned the efficacy of many of the measures used to control public behaviour. One of their studies investigated the "loss aversion" construct that was introduced earlier in this book. This construct is built on the premise that people tend to attach more value to losses than to gains if both are judged to be about the same size. In the context of the pandemic therefore it would be expected that any messages that emphasise lives lost to COVID-19 are likely to carry more weight than messages about interventions that would save the same number of lives. At least, this is the outcome that would have been expected from previous research not about the pandemic.

The researchers from Kings College tested this hypothesis by randomly assigning a sample of 500 people to two different conditions in which they were presented with one of two messages. One of these talked about lives lost and the other about lives saved by specific actions (Sanders et al., 2021). The gain frame stated that as many 100,000 people could be saved by a well-managed extension to the lockdown. The loss frame stated that the same number of lives could be saved by the same action.

All participants were then asked to say how long they thought the lockdown should last for schools, offices and different types of business. They are also asked about their intentions to comply with various government advisories and guidelines such as handwashing and social distancing.

In this study, those participants exposed to the lives lost message were not more cautious about ending lockdown than those exposed to the lives saved message. Previous research would have predicted that the first message might have had this impact. Nor were those shown the loss message more likely to comply with government behavioural recommendations. It is possible that the research took place after acceptance of death tolls was embedded in the psyches of participants and so they did not have the impact they might have had at an earlier point in the pandemic when these figures may have had more shock value. Furthermore, by the time the research was conducted many people had already died and as the death toll eased off, the "loss value" of this factor could have weakened because it had already happened. More often, in nudge experiments, participants make choices on the basis of anticipated future events and outcomes.

Another study tried to measure the effects of a number of different nudges deployed between April and June 2020 during the first UK lockdown. The nudges in question seemed to have some impact on public awareness of what they should do but they did not have a strong impact upon eventual behaviour change (Hume et al., 2021).

This study again constructed a simulated pandemic messaging scenario. The people taking part were assigned to three conditions in which they were presented with different online news articles about coronavirus. One nudge message reported that large numbers of people were being compliant with lockdown restrictions. Another message talked about an older person who was especially at risk and therefore unable to leave their home for their own safety. The researchers noted that when positive public behaviour is highlighted this can encourage others to follow suit if they are inspired to do so by such stories. People might also judge that there would be personal benefits of value to be gained in this way. The final message simply talked in general terms about how everyone could take steps to maintain their physical and mental health during the pandemic. This was treated as a control or "non-nudge" condition.

In another twist to this experiment, some participants were invited to think about someone they knew who was likely to be seriously affected by the pandemic and to produce a brief written description of the steps this person was taking to cope with the pandemic. This was regarded as a further "nudge" in terms of getting participants to consider their own behaviour. All participants were then asked to indicate their own intentions to stay at home (or not) over the next five days and their intentions in regard to compliance with a number of other COVID-19 guidelines.

The findings showed that those participants in the nudge conditions, in terms of the messages to which they were exposed (i.e., messages one and two) and in terms of whether they had been encouraged to think about someone they knew, expressed stronger intentions to comply with public health guidelines. When follow-up exercises were carried out with the same participants one to two weeks later, these intentions among the nudged had become significantly weaker. Indeed, the "nudged" were no more likely to say they would comply than the "non-nudged".

Hard and Soft Nudges

There is an important distinction to be made between two broad types of nudges, classified as System 1 and System 2. System 1 nudges use direct warnings and signage to instruct people in behaviour change. Hence, entry into a shop or restaurant may require people to wear a face mask. Hand sanitiser is visibly present upon initial entry and encourages people to clean their hands. System 2 nudges are more subtle and are grounded in the provision factual disclosures and statistical information that encourage people to make their own judgements about their behaviour often based on estimates of personal risks (Felsen et al., 2013; Hansen & Jespersen, 2013).

System 1 nudges are overt and play to deliberate decision making. In other words, they issue dos and don'ts in terms of behaviour and command public compliance. System 2 nudges invite people to calculate their own risks on the basis of relevant factual information. It is more covert in nature in that System 2 influences do not flow from deliberate instructions about how to behave. It relies on educating people and presenting cautionary advice that they are invited to consider in making up their own minds about how to behave. The hope is that people will make the judgements authorities are looking for. In that regard, nudge messages can be manipulated to emphasise specific outcomes over others in the knowledge, for example, outcomes that suggest losses to people will generally be given more weight than outcomes that bring benefits.

Value judgements might also feature within the context of nudges. This means that people are invited to make choices that represent "the right thing to do" perhaps because they will benefit others as well as being in their own best interests. These "pro-social" nudges have been found to provide encouragement to many people to follow the lead being set by authorities, for example, in the context of a health emergency or objective (Hagman et al., 2015; Junghans et al., 2015; Reisch et al., 2017). Nudges that make appeals to the "collective interest" in this way as opposed to the "individual interest" can often work well in collectivistic societies (Pe'er et al., 2019; Sunstein et al., 2018, 2019). In more individualistic societies these kinds of nudge approaches can still work, but they end to meet with less enthusiasm (Reisch et al., 2017).

In the Far East, where collectivistic societies prevail, research showed that nudge approaches that appealed to the public good proved to be effective in encouraging people to change their behaviour patterns to avoid crowded places and not meet up with close social contacts during the COVID-19 pandemic (Guan et al., 2021; Moriwaki et al., 2020; Prasetyo & Sofyan, 2020). Elsewhere, similar approaches discourage people from making long trips to celebrate religious festivals during the pandemic (Prasetyo & Sofyan, 2020).

In contrast to these findings, other studies reported more mixed success in changing public behaviour via nudge approaches. In one study, System 2 nudges designed to enhance compliance with pandemic-related restrictions failed to achieve that outcome but did increase concern about COVID-19 among young adults in Colombia (Blackman & Hoffman, 2021). In the United States, classed as an individualistic society, the significance of culture to how people responded to specific appeals again became apparent. American people exhibited greater attention on social media to messages such as "protect yourself" or "protect your loved ones" than to an appeal couched in terms of "protecting your community" (Banker & Park, 2020). In showing also how the developmental context of a pandemic, in which transmission rates and death rates, and associate risk perceptions, can change over time, some weeks later, a community-level appeal did prove to be effective in encouraging people to wear face masks (Capraro & Barcelo, 2020).

What lessons can be learned from this? Nudges can be useful mechanisms for encouraging public change under the right circumstances. Choosing the right nudges for the occasion is also important. Nudges can be explicit or implicit. They can take the form of "hard" rules and take on the form of commands. The risk here for behaviour change policy makers is that these harder nudges can trigger psychological reactance among some sectors of the public who simply reject these instructions because they can or because they simply do not like being told what to do. Soft nudges are more subtle and comprise information campaigns that are far less explicit in form and content. The public is fed factual or statistical information which invite them to weigh up odds of different outcomes for themselves and others of specific behavioural habits or patterns. They are not told what to do but they are invited to make personal judgements about specific issues by having their attention drawn to them. Governments and other authorities can still manipulate behaviour choices and outcomes by selectively feeding information designed to push or "nudge" people towards specific decisions.

As the UK government learned during the early phase of the pandemic, going subtle might not be drastic enough to procure the kinds of extreme behaviour changes needed to slow the spread of a mostly airborne disease (Sibony, 2020). Taking a harder approach risked push-back from the public, but by compulsory closures of most physical spaces in which people could meet, they gave the British public few options in terms of non-compliance. Softer nudges that continued in the form of regular televised briefings in which much of the time was spent emphasising rising infection, hospitalisation and death rates, the public was repeatedly primed to consider personal risks and these rose so too did fear of infection.

Stories that abounded within the mainstream media about celebrities and public figures, including several senior government members and their senior advisors who had succumbed to COVID-19, brought home the fact that the coronavirus did not discriminate in terms of who it infected. When the UK's Prime Minister was admitted to intensive care after struggling to stay at work for a week with the illness and came close to death, people across the country realised how serious COVID-19 could get. These unanticipated "nudges" would have helped to encourage public compliance with pandemic-related restrictions even though they had meant for many people suspending their normal lives.

One of the key factors at play psychologically in this context was public risk perception. As research in other contexts such as climate change and combatting terrorism has suggested, public support for restrictive policies and behaviour change can be motivated once people have recognised the risks of non-compliance (Drews et al., 2016; Liu et al., 2019; Zahran et al., 2006). More evidence is needed to understand the role played by risk perception in relation to the effectiveness of nudging. Early evidence has suggested that it is a factor that can make a difference (Bates et al., 2018; Sunstein et al., 2019).

As the pandemic wore on and restrictions in many countries were relaxed only later to be tightened again as COVID-19 re-surfaced once people started to interact more, hard nudges were again needed to counter public fatigue with having their lives put on hold for an, as yet, undefined period.

In a Hungarian study, the impact of nudges or regulations was investigated in relation to encouraging people to adopt preventive behaviours such as physical distancing, handwashing and wearing face masks. In general, the Hungarian public supported the use of these measures and no evidence emerged that nudging approaches had been any more effective than restrictive regulations. People who felt most at risk supported both policies and, if anything, slightly preferred regulations over nudges. Those feeling most at risk had often either had the disease themselves or knew someone such as a family member or close friend who had been infected. Yet, those who had been infected themselves were less likely to support restrictive regulations, but they supported both nudge policies and regulations if a loved one had caught COVID-19 (Dudás & Szántó, 2021). This study therefore indicated that nudges worked well in relation to some behaviour changes and not so well for others. Such evidence nonetheless points the way towards other research that can target these subtleties of nudging impacts to tease out when it could be useful and when not.

One interesting lesson learned from this research was that people who had been infected with COVID-19 and then recovered might push back harder than most against further restrictions on their everyday behaviours perhaps because they feel they are now immune and therefore no longer need to take precautions for personal safety reasons. Yet, a valid rationale for even these individuals to accept further behavioural restrictions might still exist because they could still become and then spread it to others. Whether this reasoning would carry weight with them will depend upon how collectivistic rather than individualistic they feel.

References

Asimakopoulou, K. (2020). Unrealistic optimism is fuelling the burning building. *BMJ*, 368: m1101. Retrieved from: https://www.bmj.com/content/368/bmj.m1101/rr-6

Asimakopoulou, K., Hoorens, V., Speed, E., Coulson, N. S., Antoniszczak, D., Collyer, F., Deschrijver, E., Dubbin, L., Faulks, D., Forsyth, R., Goltsi, V., Harsløf, I., Larsen, K., Manaras, I., Olczak-Kowalczyk, D., Willis, K., Xenou, T., & Scambler, S. (2020). Comparative optimism about infection and recovery from COVID-19; Implications for adherence with lockdown advice. *Health Expectations*, 23(6):1502–1511. https://doi.org/10.1111/hex.13134

Asimakopoulou, K. G., Skinner, T. C., Spimpolo, J., Marsh, S., & Fox, C. (2008). Unrealistic pessimism about risk of coronary heart disease and stroke in patients with type 2 diabetes. *Patient Education Counselling*, 71: 95–101.

Banker, S., & Park, J. (2020). Evaluating prosocial COVID-19 messaging frames: Evidence from a field study on Facebook. *Judgment and Decision Making*, 15(6), 1037–1043.

Bates, S., Holmes, J., Gavens, L., de Matos, E. G., Li, J., Ward, B., et al. (2018). Awareness of alcohol as a risk factor for cancer is associated with public support for alcohol policies. *BMC Public Health*, 18, Article number: 688. https://doi.org/10.1186/s12889-018-5581-8

Bavel, J. J. V. et al. (2020). Using social and behavioural science to support COVID-19 pandemic response. *Nature and Human Behaviour*, 4(5), 460–471. doi: 10.1038/s41562-020-0884-z

Benartzi, S., Beshears, J., Milkman, K. L., Sunstein, C. R., Thaler, R. H., Shankar, M., et al. (2017). Should governments invest more in nudging? *Psychological Science*, 28(8), 1041–1055.

Bish, A., & Michie, S. (2010). Demographic and attitudinal determinants of protective behaviours during a pandemic: A review. *British Journal of Health Psychology*, 15(pt 4), 797–824.

Blackman, A., & Hoffmann, B. (2021). Prevention among Colombian young adults. IDB Working Paper. Diminishing Returns: Nudging Covid-19 Series: 2021–1217. Retrieved from: https://publications.iadb.org/publications/english/document/Diminishing-Returns-Nudging-Covid-19-Prevention-Among-Colombian-Young-Adults.pdf

Burger, J. M., & Burns, L. (1988). The illusion of unique invulnerability and the use of effective contraception. *Personality and Social Psychology Bulletin*, *14*(2), 264–270. https://doi.org/10.1177/0146167288142005

Capraro, V., & Barcelo, H. (2020). The effect of messaging and gender on intentions to wear a face covering to slow down COVID-19 transmission. *Journal of Behavioral Economics for Policy*, *4*(S2), 45–55.

Carroll, P., Sweeny, K., & Shepperd, J. A. (2006). Forsaking optimism. *Reviews of General Psychology*, *10*, 56–73.

Chambers, J. R., Windschitl, P. D., & Suls, J. (2003). Egocentrism, event frequency, and comparative optimism: When what happens frequently is "more likely to happen to me". *Personality and Social Psychology Bulletin*, *29*, 1343–1356.

Curtis, C. (2020). *COVID-19 lockdown: The public want gradual exit that prioritises economy*. London, UK: YouGov. Retrieved from: https://yougov.co.uk/topics/politics/articles-reports/2020/04/21/covid-19-lockdown-public-want-gradual-exit-priorit

Davidson, T. (2020, 3rd April). Cheltenham defends festival going ahead after racegoers report Covid-19 symptoms. *The Mirro*. Retrieved from: https://www.mirror.co.uk/news/uk-news/cheltenham-defends-festival-going-ahead-21807262

Diepeveen, S., Ling, T., Suhrcke, M., Roland, M., & Marteau, T. M. (2013). Public acceptability of government intervention to change health-related behaviours: a systematic review and narrative synthesis. *BMC Public Health*, *13*(1), 756. https://doi.org/10.1186/1471-2458-13-756

Drews, S., Bergh, J. C., & Mvd, J. (2016). What explains public support for climate policies? A review of empirical and experimental studies. *Climate Policy*, *16*(7), 855–876.

Dryhurst, S., Schneider, C. R., Kerr, J., Freeman, A. L. J., Recchia, G., van der Bles, A. M., Spiegelhalter, D., & van der Linden, S. (2020). Risk perceptions of COVID-19 around the world. *Journal of Risk Research*. https://doi.org/10.1080/13669877.2020.1758193

Dudás, L., & Szántó, R. (2021). Nudging in the time of coronavirus? Comparing public support for soft and hard preventive measures, highlighting the role of risk perception and experience. *PLoS One*, *16*(8), e0256241. https://doi.org/10.1371/journal.pone.0256241

Duffy, R. (2020). *Life Under Lockdown: Coronavirus in the UK* (65 pp.). London, UK: The Policy Institute King's College London and Ipsos Mori. Retrieved from: https://www.kcl.ac.uk/policy-institute/assets/coronavirus-in-the-uk.pdf

Farrell, C., Towle, A., & Godolphin, W. (2006). *Where's the Patient's Voice in Health Professional Education?* Vancouver, BC: University of British Columbia.

Felsen, G., Castelo, N., & Reiner, P. B. (2013). Decisional enhancement and autonomy: Public attitudes towards overt and covert nudges. *Judgment and Decision Making*, *8*(3), 202.

Guan, B., Bao, G., Liu, Q., & Raymond, R. G. (2021). Two-way risk communication, public value consensus, and citizens' policy compliance willingness about COVID-19: Multilevel analysis based on nudge view. *Administration & Society*, *53*(7), 1106–1149. https://doi.org/10.1177/0095399721990332

Hagman, W., Andersson, D., Västfjäll, D., & Tinghög, G. (2015). Public views on policies involving nudges. *Review of Philosophy and Psychology*, *6*(3), 439–453.

Hagmann, D., Siegrist, M., & Hartmann, C. (2018). Taxes, labels, or nudges? Public acceptance of various interventions designed to reduce sugar intake. *Food Policy*, *79*, 156–165.

Haigh, M. S., & List, J. A. (2005). Do professional traders exhibit myopic loss aversion? An experimental analysis. *The Journal of Finance*, *60*(1), 523–534.

Hansen, P. G., & Jespersen, A. M. (2013). Nudge and the manipulation of choice: A framework for the responsible use of the nudge approach to behaviour change in public policy. *European Journal of Risk Regulation*, *4*(1), 3–28.

Harris, P. R., Griffin, D. W., & Murray, S. (2008). Testing the limits of optimistic bias: Event and person moderators in a multilevel framework. *Journal of Personality and Social Psychology*, *95*, 1225–1237.

Hoeben, E. M., Bernasco, W., Suonperä, L. L., van Baak, C., & Rosenkrantz L. M. (2021). Social distancing compliance: A video observational analysis. *PLoS One*, *16*(3), e0248221. https://doi.org/10.1371/journal.pone.0248221

Hoorens, V. (2008). Unrealistic optimism in health and safety risks. In D. R. Rutter & L. Quine (Eds.), *Social Psychology and Health: European Perspectives* (pp. 153–174). Aldershot, UK: Ashgate.

Hoorens, V., Smits, T., & Shepperd, J. (2007). Comparative optimism in the spontaneous generation of future life-events. *British Journal of Social Psychology*, *47*, 441–451.

Hume, S., John, P., Sanders, M., & Stockdale, E. (2021). Nudge in the time of coronavirus: The compliance to behavioural messages during crisis (20th March). Available at: https://ssrn.com/abstract=3644165 or 10.2139/ssrn.3644165

Jang, W. M., Jang, D. H., & Lee, J. Y. (2020). Social distancing and transmission-reducing practices during the 2019 coronavirus disease and 2015 Middle East Respiratory Syndrome coronavirus outbreaks in Korea. *Journal of Korean Medical Science*, *35*(23), e220. https://doi.org/10.3346/jkms.2020.35.e220

Jung, J. Y., & Mellers, B. A. (2016). American attitudes toward nudges. *Judgment and Decision Making*, *11*(1), 62–74.

Junghans, A. F., Cheung, T. T., & De Ridder, D. D. (2015). Under consumers' scrutiny—an investigation into consumers' attitudes and concerns about nudging in the realm of health behavior. *BMC Public Health*, *15*(1), 336.

Kings College London. (2020, 13th October). Perception of risk and optimism barriers in behaviour during coronavirus. *Science Daily*. Retrieved from: https://www.sciencedaily.com/releases/2020/10/201013124116.htm

Klein, C. (2020, 15th March). Social psychology of the coronavirus: Will flies save us? *The Psychologist*. Retrieved from: https://thepsychologist.bps.org.uk/social-psychology-coronavirus-will-flies-save-us

Klein, C. T. F., & Helweg-Larsen, M. (2002). Perceived control and the optimistic bias: A meta-analytic review. *Psychology and Health*, *17*, 437–446.

Liu, H., Chen, C., Cruz-Cano, R., Guida, J. L., & Lee, M. (2021). Public compliance with social distancing measures and SARS-CoV-2 spread: A quantitative analysis of 5 states. *Public Health Reports*, *136*(4), 475–482. https://doi.org/10.1177/00333549211011254

Liu, X., Mumpower, J. L., Portney, K. E., & Vedlitz, A. (2019). Perceived risk of terrorism and policy preferences for government counterterrorism spending:

Evidence from a U.S. national panel survey. *Risk, Hazards & Crisis in Public Policy, 10*(1), 102–135.

Moriwaki, D., Harada, S., Schneider, J., & Hoshino, T. (2020). Nudging preventive behaviors in COVID-19 crisis: A large scale RCT using smartphone/advertising. Institute for Economics Studies, Keio University, 2020-021. Available from: https://ideas.repec.org/p/keo/dpaper/2020-021.html

Mortimer, H. (2020, 30th April). Coronavirus: Cheltenham festival 'may have accelerated' spread. *BBC News.* Retrieved from: https://www.bbc.co.uk/news/uk-england-gloucestershire-52485584

Pe'er, E., Feldman, Y., Gamliel, E., Sahar, L., Tikotsky, A., Hod, N., et al. (2019). Do minorities like nudges? The role of group norms in attitudes towards behavioral policy. *Judgment and Decision Making, 14*(1), 40–50.

Prasetyo, D. B., & Sofyan, L. (2020). Altering intention to Mudik during COVID-19 Pandemic: A salient cue and simple reminder treatment. https://doi.org/10.1177/0971333621990459

Radcliffe, N. M., & Klein, W. M. P. (2002). Dispositional, unrealistic, and comparative optimism: Differential relations with the knowledge and processing of risk information and beliefs about personal risk. *Personality and Social Psychology Bulletin, 28*, 836–846.

Reisch, L. A., Sunstein, C. R., & Gwozdz, W. (2017). Viewpoint: Beyond carrots and sticks: Europeans support health nudges. *Food Policy, 69*, 1–10.

Reynolds, J. P., Pilling, M., & Marteau, T. M. (2018). Communicating quantitative evidence of policy effectiveness and support for the policy: Three experimental studies. *Social Science & Medicine, 218*, 1–12.

Rothman, A. J., & Salovey, P. (1997). Shaping perceptions to motivate healthy behavior: The role of message framing. *Psychological bulletin, 121*(1), 3.

Rudisill, C. (2013). How do we handle new health risks? Risk perception, optimism, and behaviors regarding the H1N1 virus. *Journal of Risk Research, 16*(8), 959–980. https://doi.org/10.1080/13669877.2012.761271

Ruthig, J. C., Chipperfield, J. G., Perry, R. P., Newall, N. E., Newall, N. E., & Swift, A. (2007). Comparative risk and perceived control: Implications for psychological and physical well-being among older adults. *Journal of Social Psychology, 147*, 345–369.

Sanders, M., Stockdale, E., Hume, S., & John, P. (2021). Loss aversion fails to replicate in the coronavirus pandemic: Evidence from an online experiment. *Economic Letters, 199*, 109433. https://doi.org/10.1016/j.econlet.2020.109433

Shepperd, J. A., Findley-Klein, C., Kwavnick, K. D., Walker, D., & Perez, S. (2000). Bracing for loss. *Journal of Personality and Social Psychology, 78*, 620–634.

Sibony, A. L. (2020). The UK COVID-19 response: A behavioural irony? *European Journal of Risk Regulation, 11*(2), 350–357.

Siedner, M. J., Harling, G., Reynolds, Z., Gilbert, R. F., Haneuse, S., Venkataramani, A. S., & Tsai, A. C. (2020). Social distancing to slow the US COVID-19 epidemic: Longitudinal pretest-posttest comparison group study. *PLoS Medicine, 17*(8), e1003244. https://doi.org/10.1371/journal.pmed.1003244

Slovic, P., Finucane, M. L., Peters, E., & MacGregor, D. G. (2004). Risk as analysis and risk as feelings: Some thoughts about affect, reason, risk, and rationality. *Risk Anal, 24*, 311–322.

Sunstein, C. R. (2016). People prefer System 2 nudges (kind of). *Duke LJ, 66*, 121–168.

Sunstein, C. R., Reisch, L. A., & Kaiser, M. (2019). Trusting nudges? Lessons from an international survey. *Journal of European Public Policy, 26*(10), 1417–1443.

Sunstein, C. R., Reisch, L. A., & Rauber, J. (2018). A worldwide consensus on nudging? Not quite, but almost. *Regulation & Governance, 12*(1), 3–22.

Taylor, S. E., & Brown, J. D. (1988). Illusion and well-being: A social psychological perspective on mental health. *Psychol Bull, 103*, 193–210.

Taylor, S. F., & Brown, J. D. (1994). Positive illusions and well-being revisited: Separating fact from fiction. *Psychological Bulletin, 116*, 21–27.

Thaler, R. H., & Sunstein, C. R. (2008). *Nudge: Improving Decisions about Health, Wealth, and Happiness.* New Haven, Conn: Yale University Press.

Trope, Y., & Liberman, N. (2010). Construal theory. *Psychological Review, 117*(2), 440–463.

Tversky, A., & Kahneman, D. (1973). Availability: A heuristic for judging frequency and probability. *Cognitive Psychology, 5*(2), 207–232.

Tversky, A., & Kahneman, D. (1979). Prospect theory: An analysis of decision under risk. *Econometrica, 47*(2), 263–291.

van der Linden, S. (2014). On the relationship between personal experience, affect and risk perception: The case of climate change. *European Journal of Social Psychology, 44*(5), 430–440.

van der Linden, S. (2015). The social-psychological determinants of climate change risk perceptions: Towards a comprehensive model. *Journal of Environmental Psychology, 41*, 112–124.

Weber, E. U. (2006). Experience-based and description-based perceptions of long-term risk: Why global warming does not scare us (yet). *Climatic Change, 77*(1/2), 103–120.

Weinstein, N. D. (1980). Unrealistic optimism about future life events. *Journal of Personality and Social Psychology, 39*, 806–820.

Wise, T., Zbozinek, T. D., Michelini, G., Hagan, C. C., & Mobbs, D. (2020). In risk perception and protective behavior during the first week of the COVID-19 pandemic in the United States. Preprint at *PsyArXiv.* https://osf.io/dz428

Wood, G., & Carroll, R. (2020, 2nd April). Cheltenham faces criticism after racegoers suffer Covid-19 symptoms. *The Guardian.* Retrieved from: https://www.theguardian.com/sport/2020/apr/02/cheltenham-faces-criticism-after-racegoers-suffer-covid-19-symptoms

Zahran, S., Brody, S. D., Grover, H., & Vedlitz, A. (2006). Climate change vulnerability and policy support. *Society & Natural Resources, 19*(9), 771–789.

Chapter 7

Social Identity, Group Processes and Physical Distancing

There was a presumption in the pre-lockdown phase of the COVID-19 pandemic that the public could not be expected to accept widespread restrictions on their everyday activities. Even if they did so at the outset, they would quickly grow tired of being told what to do. In practice, what happened when severe restrictions were imposed on public behaviour was that most people accepted these interventions, understood why they were necessary and complied. Of course, it is possible that for some people, there was an expectation that although it was necessary to take wide-ranging steps to bring a rapidly spreading airborne virus under control, there was a hope that lockdown of society would be temporary. In this context, "temporary" meant a few months (LSE, 2020).

Psychologists argued that the reaction of people around the world should not have been seen as surprising. Even in open liberal democracies in which people expect to enjoy considerable freedom of action and therefore might be expected to rebel against constraints on their normal activities, most people played along. Understanding how the public would react to specific advice, recommendations and behaviour changes, especially over time, was a more complex affair. As the experience of hindsight showed, when an intervention such as vaccination was finally developed and approved for use, and found to be effective, not everyone accepted this new protection with enthusiasm. Some people rejected COVID-19 vaccines and refused to get jabbed. A similar division in acceptance and compliance occurred in respect of wearing face masks. Not everyone complied with this behaviour.

In these cases, the reasons for differences in people's opinions and behaviour could be explained at least in part in terms of social group dynamics. People did not just listen to the advice of their government or of the government's chief medical and scientific advisers, they also referred to groups to which they belonged or aspired to join. If such groups advised against following the government's rulebook, individuals would follow the lead of their key reference groups. Understanding behavioural compliance with pandemic-related restrictions therefore needed to be informed by these group dynamics (Drury et al., 2020).

DOI: 10.4324/9781003274308-7

The public's assessment of risk was recognised as a key component of people's decision making during the pandemic. There was little doubt that governments and public health authorities used informational techniques and messages that were designed to highlight risks. This represented part of a mixture of ingredients of communications strategies geared to manipulating public behaviour. Whether or not people invariably accepted whatever their government told them was debatable. There were indications from many countries that they did. Often, people had no choice because many of the spaces in which they would perform normal activities were either closed down or had compulsory restrictions imposed upon them in terms of how people could behave. In addition, there were other advisories concerning people's behaviours that could only work with the full cooperation of the public.

One of the factors that could mediate the public's acceptance of government advisories and their willingness voluntarily to comply with them was their perceptions of how other people behaved. In particular, people who belonged to the same social groups could be an especially significant point of reference in this context. Following key premises of the social identity model, people's behaviours were expected to follow the lead of their reference and membership groups. If fellow group members were inclined to follow government advice, the probability that others in the group would follow suit. People's actions were already known to be guided by social norms (Smith, 2020).

A Group Processes and Social Identity Perspective

A group processes perspective to investigating and understanding how people respond to major crises and emergencies has proven useful because it can offer varying interpretations of public behaviour that can explain propensities either to respond to risks or not to do so when expected. In a context such as that presented by the COVID-19 pandemic, early public compliance with severe restrictions on their normal everyday behaviours was sometimes explained in terms of risk avoidance. Constant daily reports of death rates from COVID-19 drew extra attention to worst-case outcomes that in terms of their statistical probability only affected a small minority of all people. Yet, this was not the impression created by round-the-clock news reporting on the pandemic.

Although many people perceived the risks of COVID-19, perhaps to an exaggerated degree, and experienced accompanying fear and threat responses, others did not. When protective measures such as wearing face masks and getting vaccinated were widely promoted, many people took advantage of these interventions, and others did not. Why did these different reactions occur? One explanation that derives from a groups processes and social identity perspective is that people do not rely solely on the advice of government or experts or the media. They also listen to other sources and often these are social groups to which they belong. Complying with the advice or the perspective of these groups can outweigh the influence of the authorities. This can lead some people therefore to behave differently from the recommendations or requirements of their governments (Drury et al., 2020).

There are occasions when reference groups encourage people to behave more compliantly with government requests and even to go beyond the action government advises everyone to take. Then, there are times when reference groups' perspectives conflict with the requests of the authorities.

Individuals can potentially belong to many groups and may also aspire to join many others. These membership and reference groups serve as sources of reference for individuals when seeking guidance on how to behave in different social settings (Moscovici, 1988). Groups develop their own norms and rules concerning appropriate behavioural responses across different situations (Reicher et al., 2010). These norms can also influence the ways individuals react cognitively and emotionally to different social experiences (Neville et al., 2020; Reicher et al., 2016). Referencing back to these psychological dynamics can yield important insights into why people responded in the ways they did to the severe behavioural restrictions imposed upon them by their governments during the COVID-19 pandemic (Reicher & Stott, 2020).

Another aspect of group processes influences is social identity. This concept refers to the degree to which individuals value the norms of a membership or reference group to a point where they define the individual's own character or sense of "self" (Hornsey, 2008; Tajfel & Turner, 1979). Self-identity means not just that groups are used as reference points for seeking guidance about how to behave in specific situations, but also that some groups may be more influential than others in this context. This principle came into play in relation to people's compliance with pandemic-related advice or restrictions (Capraro & Barcelo, 2020; Levita, 2020).

Group Processes and Public Involvement in Pandemic Control

In studies of why the public behaved this way group processes were identified as playing a part. Many people recognised the need for the non-pharmaceutical interventions and many believed that these measures were effective in controlling the pandemic (Clark et al., 2020). Hence, not only were people doing as they were told, they were also working together under a fresh community spirit that emerged during the pandemic (Parveen & McIntyre, 2020). Research surfaced to show that people had created a shared sense of purpose and cooperation in playing their part in managing the crisis that had arisen with the pandemic. There was an increased sense of civic responsibility and a greater sense of caring for those who were vulnerable and most at risk (Everett et al., 2020; Goldberg et al., 2020;

Vignoles et al., 2020). This spirit of collective responsibility meant that coercion was not needed to procure the public's cooperation with new rules of behaviour (Jackson et al., 2020; Sharkey, 2020; Wolf et al., 2020).

In addition, those who chose to flout the behavioural restrictions could become targets of criticism (Prosser et al., 2020). These social group pressures to comply with the rules reinforced government restrictions and might have been more difficult for miscreants to avoid when the pressure to comply was coming from all around them (Public Health England, 2020).

Despite this community spiritedness, over time more and more people found strict compliance with all the restrictions more challenging. Evidence started to emerge as the lockdown in the United Kingdom eased in the early summer of 2020, that growing numbers of people reported less than 100% compliance (Fancourt et al., 2020b).

It could have been that behaviour fatigue was setting in. It could also have been that many people had started to recalculate the risks from COVID-19. Some may have caught the disease and come through it unscathed while others had avoided it and felt reassured therefore that perhaps they were effective in their behaviour at keeping themselves safe. Others could have been reassured also that there were mitigating factors such as wearing face masks that meant it was safe for them to venture out of their homes more frequently and to enter spaces where they would meet with others at minimal risk. As the infection rates fell away in the summer months, people might have been further reassured by the significantly reduced circulation of the virus which meant that they were less and less likely to bump into infected people (ONS, 2020a, 2020b).

Ingroup versus Outgroup Influences

A series of experiments in the United Kingdom confirmed that "ingroup" members were important reference sources for individuals who had not yet decided how to behave. Individuals would follow the lead set by influential reference group members in whom they placed considerable trust. Individuals would also find those sources to be more credible. If reference groups put out a different message about risk from that of the government, the likelihood that government advice would be followed diminished (Cruwys et al., 2021).

The significance of group processes and social identity was evidenced in a study in the United States which surveyed people about their face-mask-wearing behaviour and physical distancing. Comparing across 12 states, adoption of these precautionary and protective behaviours was higher in states where people were generally more oriented towards trying to control the transmission of COVID-19 and occurred independently of state government mandates concerning these behaviours. This meant that there was a stronger and positive community orientation towards adopting these behaviours which encouraged people to comply (Rader et al., 2021).

A further finding in relation to group influences is that people will tend to take more risks with members of an ingroup than with outgroup members. This behaviour pattern is linked to the relative degrees of trust individuals place in others that will also depend upon their familiarity with others and perceptions of similarities with themselves. This tendency can have both good and bad consequences. If ingroup encourage individuals to take un-necessary risks, their influences will often not be beneficial.

Research in the United Kingdom and Australia found that people who identified with their neighbours tended also to trust them more. Willingness to get vaccinated was strengthened and perceived risks associated with it weakened when vaccination was endorsed by an ingroup member (Cruwys, Stevens et al., 2021).

The adoption of preventive behaviours depended on a range of factors. Among these were fear of COVID-19 and trust in information sources. Greater fear and greater trust were significantly associated with greater adoption of precautionary behaviours. In predictive modelling, these two variables accounted for over a quarter (27%) of the variance in prevention behaviour. Countering these effects, at least indirectly was the propensity to believe conspiracy theories about the coronavirus. As scepticism about the pandemic and their government's attempts to bring it under control grew, the less people felt threatened by the pandemic and the less they trusted COVID-19 information sources (Šuriņa et al., 2021).

Social identity can influence the way the members of one group react when one of their members exhibits a breach of trust with a second group in the way they behave towards that group. When the other group displayed anger and disappointment, the ingroup member in the study was more likely to experience guilt and shame about their own group and would seek to compensate the other group when subsequently given an opportunity to do so. Similar responses occurred when the guilty ingroup member was sorry for their behaviour, but the participant in the study also felt happier that their misbehaving group member had owned up (Shore et al., 2019).

People tend to trust other people when the information about them en-ables them to judge the other's character. When this information is missing, they will use other clues, such as information about a social group to which the other person belongs. If the individual finds out that they both have membership of this social category or group in common, their trust in the other person will be strengthened (Tanis & Postmes, 2005).

Message Confusion, Behavioural Hypocrisy and Trust in Authorities

For a social group or organisation to retain the trust of its members during times of crisis, there must be a perception that those in charge seem to know what they are doing and can communicate their decisions in a clear and digestible manner. Experiences in the United Kingdom in the first phases of the pandemic served to illustrate this point. As the UK government started to change its rules and its slogans, some public confusion occurred at this time with people being unsure about what they should or should not be doing (Fancourt et al., 2020c). Such confusion converted into questions of competence and trust among growing sectors of the British public.

As more physical spaces opened again for business, such as bars, cafes, restaurants, galleries, museums, hotels, barbers/hairdressers and non-essential shops, people again got used to interpersonal contact. As confidence grew, individuals' diligence in adhering to the remaining physical distancing restrictions often relaxed (Fancourt et al., 2020a; ONS, 2020a). The community spirit and more especially a renewed sense of national identity triggered by the national lockdown, which affected everyone, also showed signs of weakening as life began to return to normal (Duffy & Allington, 2020).

Public commitment to its government's restrictions was damaged by the failure of some senior members of government, other members of parliament and senior government advisers to adhere to the rule themselves (Stewart, 2020). The highest-profile case was that of Dominic Cummings, the prime minister's senior adviser. Cummings had travelled with his wife and children to stay in close proximity to his family in the north-east of England after displaying COVID-19 symptoms in direct contravention of prevailing lockdown restrictions. While in Durham, visiting his parents, he was seen driving out with his family to visit other sites in the area, again flouting lockdown restrictions. He argued differently and claimed that technically he had not broken any laws, but at one point, Durham police challenged this position (Dodd, 2020).

Before returning to London, he took a "short drive" to Barnard Castle 30 miles away from where he was staying, accompanied by his wife and child. He explained this as an opportunity to test his eyesight to see if he was well enough to undertake the much longer drive back down to London. Many MPs, including from his own party, felt that Mr Cummings should lose his job over this behaviour. Social isolation was requirement for anyone displaying symptoms characteristic of COVID-19, but this was achieved by consent. It was felt by many MPs that his behaviour, while technically not illegal, clearly defied the spirit of the civic duty expectations being placed on every UK citizen if they thought they had caught the disease (see Child, 2020).

Before the Cummings' episode, Dr Catherine Calderwood, Scotland's chief medical officer was also forced to resign only three weeks into lockdown after being seen visiting a second home in East Fife more than an hour's drive from her main home in Edinburgh. She had been seen doing this on two separate occasions despite fronting media advertising campaigns telling everyone else to do the opposite, namely stay home and not make unnecessary trips to other places (BBC News, 2020).

The Housing, Communities and Local Government Secretary, Robert Jenrick, found himself in hot water when he travelled for over an hour to visit his parents, again directly flouting lockdown travel and home visiting rules. He drove more than 150 miles from his family home in Herefordshire to his parent's home in Shropshire. He apologised and survived public and opposition political pressure to resign (ITV News, 2020).

Another senior scientific adviser, member of SAGE (the UK government's Senior Advisory Group for Emergencies) and the architect of epidemiological research that persuaded the UK's government to go into lockdown, Professor Neil Ferguson, was found out when he allowed his married lover to visit him at his home, directly contravening government advice that people from different households should not mix. Ferguson apologised for his lack of judgement and resigned from his position on SAGE.

Scottish National Party MP, Margaret Ferrier travelled by train from Scotland to Westminster despite experiencing COVID-19 symptoms and then travelled home again after being tested and found to be positive for the virus. Although suspended by her party, Ferrier continued to serve as an independent MP and was not sacked from parliament (BBC News, 2020, 2nd October).

Although the two medical/scientific advisers resigned from their positions, most of these rule-breakers survived unscathed. This sent a message to the public that there was one rule for them and another for their national leaders (Fancourt et al., 2020d). This behaviour by those in positions of influence and power led to anger among some people who questioned why they should follow the rules themselves but for others, it made them even more determined to show they were better than those giving advice or taking decisions (Jackson et al., 2020).

A study by researchers at University College London, led by Daisy Fancourt, investigated the impact of Cummings' episode on public confidence in the government and found evidence that public opinion had been damaged (Fancourt et al., 2020d). They compared the opinions of people living in England with those living in the devolved nations of Scotland and Wales. Restrictions on people living in England had been imposed by the Westminster government whereas those imposed on people living in Scotland and Wales were determined by their own devolved assemblies. One basic finding was that the reputation of the devolved governments did not change as a result of Dominic Cummings' behaviour. The same was not true of public opinion about the Westminster government.

Tracking public opinion from the start of lockdown between 21st and 23rd March 2020, the UCL research indicated that public confidence in Boris Johnson's government improved over this period through to May when it was announced that society would begin to open up again over the summer. The devolved assemblies of Scotland and Wales exhibited core caution about unlocking restrictions too soon and argued that the Westminster government's proposal to start to release the country from lockdown at that time carried risks. Public opinion towards the Conservative government wavered at this time but then stabilised until the Cumming's episode. Public confidence in central government decreased along with the willingness of people to follow the rules.

Message clarity and consistency was another area in which public confidence in government faltered Drawing upon social psychological theory within a group processes perspective, Nerlich and Jaspal (2021) argued that the ways in which COVID-19 were represented and mitigation strategies to cope with it were presented by government and scientific experts needed to be digestible and comprehensible for the public. Messaging about the pandemic should try to be non-threatening and provide clear guidance in terms of the steps people could take to play their part in helping themselves and others.

Research by Kantar with over 1,100 people living in Great Britain conducted between 9th and 15th July 2020 was one among a number of polls at that time that uncovered a lack of public confidence in the way the government was handling the COVID-19 crisis. Over half (53%) rated the government's handling of the crisis as fairly/very poor compared with four in ten (39%) that thought the crisis was being handled well. Just half the population (50%) rated the government's communication about the virus as good (Taylor, 2020).

During the pandemic, there were opportunities for new "tribes" to emerge defined, for instance, according to whether people complied with pandemic-related restrictions on their behaviour or chose not to. To follow their leaders' wishes, there needed to be a certain amount of identification between members of the public and political leaders and senior scientific advisers and spokespersons. Once that trust was lost, the command these authorities could expend to have over the public could become critically weakened, especially when asking them to suspend their normal, everyday lives, and in many cases, suffer financial hardship and psychological distress as a result. Furthermore, when the public do not trust their political leaders anyway, governments may struggle to keep a lid on the transmission of a highly infectious new disease if they cannot procure public cooperation.

People tend to trust other people when the information about them enables them to judge the other's character. When this information is missing, they will use other clues, such as information about a social group to which the other person belongs. If the individual finds out that they both have membership of this social category or group in common, their trust in the other person will be strengthened (Tanis & Postmes, 2005). If they cannot identify with another person in these terms and their behaviour causes people to assign that person to another group with which they do not identify, the ability of that person to influence others is diminished.

This psychological phenomenon provides one explanation for the persistent division in public behaviour and behaviour between people on the basis of their political allegiances, such as was observed in the United States during the pandemic. Evidence emerged that Republican-leaning counties were less inclined to observe physical distancing advice than were Democrat-leaning counties and that this propensity became more pronounced as the pandemic wore on (Gollwitzer et al., 2020; Grossman et al., 2020). Further research had indicated that political partisanship in the United States had become a significant definer of Americans' social identity (Iyengar & Krupenkin, 2019).

Public Trust Internationally: Collectivism and Individualism

The influence of membership and reference groups on pandemic-related compliance behaviour was confirmed by a number of studies. The appeal of "civic responsibility" and the use of mantras such as "we're all in this together" as motivators of public behavioural compliance can be underpinned not just by selected and narrowly defined group identities, but also by a wider worldview. Nations and their indigenous cultures around the world have been differentiated in terms of whether they are collectivistic or individualistic.

Collectivistic cultures tend to place the need to support behaviour that benefits their community above personal ambition. Individualistic cultures are characterised by attaching importance to personal drive and achievement. In one culture, the "culture" or the wider community is prioritised and in the other the progress of the individual is promoted. In effect, "collectivistic" people are more group-oriented. They also tend to be more accepting of rule-based systems. In contrast, "individualistic" people prefer systems with fewer rules and greater freedom of individual choice (Dake, 1991; Douglas & Wildavsky, 1982).

Collectivists, hypothetically, therefore might be expected to be more ready to obey restrictions imposed by their governments or other authorities if they believe this will be to the benefit of all. Individualists would be more likely to push back against such restrictions if they felt personally unfairly treated. Research carried out during the pandemic supported these theoretically expected differences in response to pandemic-related behavioural restrictions.

A study conducted in two survey waves in Switzerland found that the participants most likely to show weaker acceptance of behavioural constraints during the pandemic tended to be more distrustful of others and of authorities, regarded the risks from COVID to be low and adhered to an individualistic worldview (Siegrist & Bearth, 2021). More generally, the public were found to have been broadly tolerant of the interventions imposed upon them to control transmission of the coronavirus, but as soon as these measures had achieved their intended objectives of bringing the pandemic under control, people grew tired of the restrictions and were more likely to flout the rules. Although specific sets of interventions might continue to receive epidemiological support, public support could evaporate over time.

Trust appeared initially to be important. This had been found elsewhere in a study of people from across ten countries, but trust, as an independent variable or causal factor was often measured in a blunt fashion (Dryhurst 2020). Potentially, public trust was a heterogeneous concept and covered "trust" of different kinds and in different entities (Siegrist, 2021). Hence, the public might distrust their government or politicians and yet trust scientists advising governments. Where trust did exist, and usually this was groups-related, risk perceptions could change (reduce in severity) along with tolerance of compliance measures (becomes stronger) (Wong & Jensen, 2020).

Groups might be known to influence people's beliefs about risks and motivations to comply with pandemic-related interventions but their efficacy in these contexts rested upon how much they were trusted (Siegrist, 2021). Greater trust in specific groups could drive a stronger tendency to believe what they say and to follow the advice they give. Hence, specific kinds of "trust" were crucial components of the psychological dynamics driving compliance behaviour (Seale et al., 2020; Ye & Lyu, 2020).

Lessons Learned

The COVID-19 pandemic forced governments around the world to take drastic action to bring under control a rapidly spreading new coronavirus that could be fatal for some at-risk people. With no vaccines or proven drug treatments available for this virus at the outset of the pandemic, governments relied instead upon other measures that essentially meant many people putting their normal lives completely on hold. Once it was clinically established that this was a mostly airborne virus, the solution to its transmission was to keep people physically apart from each other. This strategy was built upon compulsory closures of physical spaces where many people interacted such as bars, cafes, restaurants, most retail outlets, leisure and entertainment venues and sports facilities, schools and universities and many workplaces. In addition, a great deal of voluntary compliance with restrictions and other behaviour advisories was requested.

In this chapter, the significance of group processes and social identity were examined in the context of driving people's willingness to comply with drastic restrictions on their everyday behaviour. Theoretically, such factors were identified as potentially important influences over public behaviour even before the pandemic. While other theories have highlighted environmental signalling, persuasive messaging, and a combination of these and other psychological factors such as personality type in relation to triggering and maintaining behaviour modification among the general public, the perspective examined in this chapter has indicated the significance of referrals to other people and especially to groups of people that have their own identity forged out of their adopted norms and rules of behaviour.

When governments or their health authorities seek to change public behaviour in a crisis situation such as the 2020–2021 coronavirus pandemic, they need to be mindful of the mediating influences of membership and reference groups. These groups might comprise families, work colleagues, demographic categories (e.g., defined by age, gender, ethnicity, geographical location), religious or political affiliations, and special interests. Hence, willingness to comply with physical distancing restrictions will be enhanced when other people from relevant reference groups also are seen to comply. Such is the importance of group processes combined with social identity that when behaviour change messages are issued, their impact will be enhanced when they request behaviour shifts that are consistent with ones acceptable to a wider group to which they belong or refer to (Neville et al., 2021).

References

BBC News. (2020, 6th April). Coronavirus: Scotland's chief medical officer resigns over lockdown trip. Retrieved from: https://www.bbc.co.uk/news/uk-scotland-52177171

BBC News. (2020, 2nd October). MP Margaret Ferrier's COVID Parliament trip 'indefensible'. Retrieved from: https://www.bbc.co.uk/news/uk-scotland-54379026

Capraro, V., & Barcelo, H. (2020). The effect of messaging and gender on intentions to wear a face covering to slow down COVID-19 transmission. *arXiv* [Preprint] *arXiv:2005.05467*. https://doi.org/10.31234/osf.io/tg7vz

Child, D. (2020, 27th May). Two-thirds of Brits think Dominic Cummings broke lockdown rules, YouGov poll finds. *Evening Standard*. Retrieved from: https://www.standard.co.uk/news/uk/yougov-poll-majority-brits-dominic-cummings-breached-lockdown-a4450831.html

Clark, C., Davila, A., Regis, M., & Kraus, S. (2020). Predictors of COVID-19 voluntary compliance behaviors: An international investigation. *Global Transitions*, 2(2), 76–82. https://doi.org/10.1016/j.glt.2020.06.003

Cruwys, T., Greenaway, K. H., Ferris, L. J., Rathbone, J. A., Saeri, A. K., Williams, E., Parker, S. L., Chang, M. X., Croft, N., Bingley, W., & Grace, L. (2021). When trust goes wrong: A social identity model of risk taking. *Journal of Personality and Social Psychology*, 120(1), 57–83. https://doi.org/10.1037/pspi0000243

Cruwys, T., Stevens, M., Donaldson, J. L., Cárdenas, D., Platow, M. J., Reynolds, K. J., & Fong, P. (2021). Perceived COVID-19 risk is attenuated by ingroup trust: Evidence from three empirical studies. *BMC Public Health*, 21(1), 869. https://doi.org/10.1186/s12889-021-10925-3

Dake, K. (1991). Orienting dispositions in the perception of risk: An analysis of contemporary worldviews and cultural biases. *Journal of Cross-Cultural Psychology*, 22, 61–82.

Dodd, V. (2020, 28th May). Dominic Cummings potentially broke lockdown rules say Durham police. *The Guardian*. Retrieved from: https://www.theguardian.com/politics/2020/may/28/dominic-cummings-potentially-broke-lockdown-rules-say-durham-police

Douglas, M., &. Wildavsky, A. (1982). *Risk and Culture: An Essay on the Selection of Technological and Environmental Dangers*. Berkeley, CA: University of California Press.

Drury, J., Carter, H., Ntontis, E., & Guven, S. T. (2020). Public behaviour in response to the COVID-19 pandemic: Understanding the role of group processes. *BJPsych Open*. 7(1), e11. https://doi.org/10.1192/bjo.2020.139

Drury, J., Reicher, S., & Stott, C. (2020). COVID-19 in context: Why do people die in emergencies? It's probably not because of collective psychology. *British Journal of Social Psychology*, *59*(3), 686–693. https://doi.org/10.1111/bjso.12393

Dryhurst, S. et al. (2020). Risk perceptions of COVID-19 around the world. *Journal of Risk Research*, *23*, 994–1006.

Duffy, B., & Allington, D. (2020). *The Trusting, the Dissenting and the Frustrated: How the UK Is Dividing as Lockdown Is Eased*. King's College London. Retrieved from: https://www.kcl.ac.uk/policy-institute/assets/how-the-uk-is-dividing-as-the-lockdown-is-eased.pdf

Everett, J. A., Colombatto, C., Chituc, V., Brady, W. J., & Crockett, M. (2020). The effectiveness of moral messages on public health behavioral intentions during the COVID-19 pandemic. *PsyArXiv* [Preprint] 2020. Retrieved from: https://psyarxiv.com/9yqs8/

Fancourt, D., Bu, F., Mak, H. W., & Steptoe, A. (2020a). *Covid-19 Social Study. Results Release 9*. University College London. https://b6bdcb03-332c-4ff9-8b9d-28f9c957493a.filesusr.com/ugd/3d9db5_cf6736fab93e4fb898d42d8668a350a6.pdf

Fancourt, D., Bu, F., Mak, H. W., & Steptoe, A. (2020b). *Covid-19 Social Study. Results Release 16*. University College London. https://b6bdcb03-332c-4ff9-8b9d-28f9c957493a.filesusr.com/ugd/3d9db5_dc64263647624fd3842e6521c186aa69.pdf

Fancourt, D., Bu, F., Mak, H. W., & Steptoe, A. (2020c). *Covid-19 Social Study. Results Release 17*. University College London. https://b6bdcb03-332c-4ff9-8b9d-28f9c957493a.filesusr.com/ugd/3d9db5_8f72d734373243f68867ad8465fb9588.pdf

Fancourt, D., Steptoe, A., & Wright, L. (2020d). The Cummings effect: politics, trust, and behaviours during the COVID-19 pandemic. *Lance*, *396*(10249), 464–465. doi: 10.1016/S0140-6736(20)31690-1

Goldberg, M., Gustafson, A., Maibach, E., van der Linden, S., Ballew, M. T., Bergquist, P., et al. (2020). Social norms motivate COVID-19 preventive behaviors. *PsyArXiv* [Preprint]. Retrieved from: https://psyarxiv.com/9whp4.

Gollwitzer, A., Martel, C., Brady, W. J., Parnamets, P., Freedman, I. J., Knowles, E. D., & Van Bavel, J. J. (2020). Partisan differences in physical distancing are linked to health outcomes during the COVID-19 pandemic. *Nature Human Behavior*, *4*, 1186–1197.

Grossman, G., Kim, S., Rexer, J. M., & Thirumpurthy, H. (2020). Political partisanship influences behavioral responses to governors' recommendations for COVID-19 prevention in the United States. *PNAS*, *117*(39), 24114–24153.

Hornsey, M. J. (2008). Social identity theory and self-categorization theory: A historical review. *Social and Personality Psychology Compass*, *2*, 204–222.

ITV News. (2020, 22nd May). The high-profile figures who have 'breached coronavirus lockdown rules'. Retrieved from: https://www.itv.com/news/2020-05-22/the-high-profile-figures-who-have-breached-lockdown-restrictions

Iyengar, S., & Krupenkin, M. (2019). Partisanship as social identity: Implications for the study of party polarization. *The Forum.* https://doi.org/10.1515/for-2018-0003

Jackson, J., Bradford, B., Yesberg, J., Hobson, Z., Kyprianides, A., Pósch, K., et al. (2020). Public compliance and COVID-19: Did Cummings damage the fight against the virus, or become a useful anti-role model? British Politics and Policy at LSE. Retrieved from: https://blogs.lse.ac.uk/politicsandpolicy/public-compliance-covid19-june/

Levita, L. (2020). *Initial research findings on the impact of COVID-19 on the wellbeing of young people aged 13 to 24 in the UK.* COVID-19 Psychological Research Consortium (C19PRC). Retrieved from: https://drive.google.com/file/d/1AOc0wCPqv2g

LSE. (2020). The lockdown and social norms: Why the UK is complying by consent rather than compulsion. *British Politics and Policy at LSE.* Retrieved from: https://blogs.lse.ac.uk/politicsandpolicy/lockdown-social-norms/

Moscovici, S. (1988). Notes towards a description of social representations. *European Journal of Social Psychology, 18*(3), 211–250.

Nerlich, B., & Jaspal, R. (2021). Social representations of 'social distancing' in response to COVID-19 in the UK media. *Current Sociology, 69*(4), https://doi.org/10.1177/0011392121990030

Neville, F. G., Novelli, D., Drury, J., & Reicher, S. (2020). Shared social identity transforms social relations in imaginary crowds. *Group Processes and Intergroup Relations.* https://doi.org/10.1177/1368430220936759

Neville, F. G., Templeton, F., Smith, J. R., & Louis, W. R. (2021). Social norms, social identities and the COVID-19 pandemic: Theory and recommendations. *Social and Personality Psychology Compass, 15*(5). https://doi.org/10.1111/spc3.12596

Office for National Statistics. (2020a). *Coronavirus and the social impacts on Great Britain: 30 April 2020.* Office for National Statistics. Retrieved from: https://www.ons.gov.uk/peoplepopulationandcommunity/healthandsocialcare/healthandwellbeing/bulletins/coronavirusandthesocialimpactsongreatbritain/30april2020#actions-undertaken-to-prevent-the-spread-of-the-coronavirus

Office for National Statistics. (2020b). *Coronavirus and the social impacts on Great Britain: 29 May 2020.* Office for National Statistics. Retrieved from: https://www.ons.gov.uk/peoplepopulationandcommunity/healthandsocialcare/healthandwellbeing/bulletins/coronavirusandthesocialimpactsongreatbritain/29may2020#actions-undertaken-to-prevent-the-spread-of-the-coronavirus

Parveen, N., & McIntyre, N. (2020). Britons think UK will be more united after coronavirus recovery. *The Guardian.* Retrieved from: https://www.theguardian.com/world/2020/may/29/britons-think-uk-will-be-more-united-after-coronavirus-recovery

Prosser, A. M., Judge, M., Bolderdijk, J. W., Blackwood, L., & Kurz, T. (2020). 'Distancers' and 'non-distancers'? The potential social psychological impact of moralizing COVID-19 mitigating practices on sustained behaviour change. *British Journal of Social Psychology, 59*(3), 653–662.

Public Health England. (2020). Disparities in the risk and outcomes of COVID-19. Public Health England. Retrieved from: https://assets.publishing.service.gov.uk/government/uploads/system/uploads/attachment_data/file/892085/disparities_review.pdf

Rader, B., White, L. F., Burns, M. R., Chen, J., Brilliant, J., Cohen, J., Shaman, J., Brilliant, L., Kraemer, M. U. G., Hawkins, J. B., Scarpino, S. V., Astley, C. M., & Brownstein, J. S. (2021). Mask-wearing and control of SARS-CoV-2 transmission in the USA: A cross-sectional study. *Lancet Digital Health*, *3*(3), e148–e157. https://doi.org/10.1016/S2589-7500(20)30293-4

Reicher, S., Spears, R., & Haslam, S. A. (2010). The social identity approach in social psychology. In M. S. Wetherell & C. T. Mohanty (Eds.), *Sage Identities Handbook* (pp. 45–62). Thousand Oaks, CA: SAGE.

Reicher, S., & Stott, C. (2020). On order and disorder during the COVID-19 pandemic. *British Journal of Social Psychology*, *59*(3), 694–702.

Reicher, S. D., Templeton, A., Neville, F., Ferrari, L., & Drury, J. (2016). Core disgust is attenuated by ingroup relations. *Proceedings of the National Academy of Sciences of the United States of America*, *113*(10), 2631–2635.

Seale, H. et al. (2020). COVID-19 is rapidly changing: Examining public perceptions and behaviors in response to this evolving pandemic. *PloS One*, *15*(6), e0235112. https://doi.org/10.1371/journal.pone.0235112

Sharkey, P. (2020). The US has a collective action problem that's larger than the coronavirus crisis. *Vox*. Retrieved from: https://www.vox.com/2020/4/10/21216216/coronavirus-social-distancing-texas-unacast-climate-change

Shore, D. M., Rychlowska, M., van der Schalk, J., Parkinson, B., & Manstead, A. S. R. (2019). Intergroup emotional exchange: Ingroup guilt and outgroup anger increase resource allocation in trust games. *Emotion*, *9*(4), 605–616. https://doi.org/10.1037/emo0000463

Siegrist, M. (2021). Trust and risk perception: A critical review of the literature. *Risk Analysis*, *41*, 480–490.

Siegrist, M., & Bearth, A. (2021). Worldviews, trust and risk perceptions shape public acceptance of COVID-19 public health measures. *Proceedings of the National Academy of Sciences of the United States of America*, *118*(24), e2100411118. https://doi.org/10.1073/pnas.2100411118

Smith, J. R. (2020). Group norms. In O. Braddick (Ed.), *Oxford Research Encyclopaedia of Psychology*. Oxford, UK: University of Oxford Press. https://doi.org/10.1093/acrefore/9780190236

Stewart, H. (2020, 5th May). Neil Ferguson: UK coronavirus adviser resigns after breaking lockdown rules. *The Guardian*. Retrieved from: https://www.theguardian.com/uk-news/2020/may/05/uk-coronavirus-adviser-prof-neil-ferguson-resigns-after-breaking-lockdown-rules

Šuriņa, S., Martinsone, K., Perepjolkina, V., Kolesnikova, J., Vainik, U., Ruža, A., Vrublevska, J., Smirnova, D., Fountoulakis, K. N., & Rancans, E. (2021). Factors related to COVID-19 preventive behaviors: A structural equation model. *Frontiers in Psychology*, *12*, 676521. https://doi.org/10.3389/fpsyg.2021.676521

Tajfel, H., & Turner, J. C. (1979). An integrative theory of intergroup conflict. In S. Worchel, & W. G. Austin (Eds.), *The Psychology of Intergroup Relations* (pp. 33–47). Pacific Grove, CA: Brooks-Cole.

Tanis, M., & Postmes, T. (2005). A social identity approach to trust: Interpersonal perception, group membership and trusting behaviour. *European Journal of Social Psychology, 35*, 413–424.

Taylor, L. (2020, 15th July). Eight in ten Brits in favour of local lockdowns to tackle coronavirus. *Kantar*. Available at: www.kantar.com/inspiration/politics/eight-in-ten-in-favour-of-local-lockdowns-to-tackle-coronavirus

Vignoles, V., Jaser, Z., Taylor, F., & Ntontis, E. (2020). Harnessing shared identities to mobilise resilient responses to the COVID-19 pandemic. *PsyArXiv* [Preprint]. Retrieved from: https://psyarxiv.com/g9q5u/

Wolf, L. J., Haddock, G., Manstead, A. S., & Maio, G. R. (2020). The importance of (shared) human values for containing the COVID-19 pandemic. *British Journal of Social Psychology, 59*(3), 618–627.

Wong, C. M. L., & Jensen, O. (2020). The paradox of trust: Perceived risk and public compliance during the COVID-19 pandemic in Singapore. *Journal of Risk Research, 23*, 1021–1030.

Ye, M., & Lyu, Z. (2020). Trust, risk perception, and COVID-19 infections: Evidence from multilevel analyses of combined original dataset in China. *Social Science and Medicine, 265*, 113517.

Chapter 8

Theory of Planned Behaviour and Physical Distancing

The theory of planned behaviour (TPB) outlines a number of internal psychological factors that can be triggered to drive behaviour change (Ajzen, 1991). The key variables that come into play are "attitudes" and "beliefs" that individuals hold about the behaviour to be changed, their perceptions of how others regard this behaviour and perform it ("subjective norms"), and finally individuals' perceptions that the behaviour change is within their scope or ability to adopt or change ("behavioural control"). When these internal factors are engaged and lined up in a positive fashion, they increase an individual's intention to adopt or change the target behaviour. The ultimate success of the model is measured in terms of whether it does accurately and effectively predict behaviour change (Ajzen & Madden, 1986; Eagly & Chaiken, 1993).

A person must have a positive attitude towards a behaviour and must believe that it will produce a positive outcome for them before being inclined to perform it. This is often not enough by itself to trigger behaviour change, but it is important to set in motion a relevant chain of internal cognitive precursors of behaviour change. What will also help is if the individual believes that the behaviour change will produce positive or beneficial end-results for them.

Individuals then turn their attention to what other people are doing. Are others showing a propensity to adopt the behaviour change? Are the actions of others important to the individual? Does this apply to people in general or to those individuals who turn to first for guidance in how to behave (e.g., reference groups). If others are compliant, then, there would be social pressure on individuals to conform with perceived population or reference group norms. This pressure will increase the probability of an individual saying that they intend to behave in that way. Even if this stacks up positively alongside internal attitudes and beliefs about the behaviour itself, this still might be enough to motivate behaviour change. The individual has to believe that the behaviour in question is feasible for them. If the behaviour is simply not possible because they believe they lack the skills to perform it or because to do so would cause unpleasant collateral side effects, then even if they believe

DOI: 10.4324/9781003274308-8

the behaviour could be worthwhile, they still would not be able to adopt it themselves (Ajzen, 2001; Ajzen & Kruglanski, 2019).

In the context of the COVID-19 pandemic, therefore, this model would enable researchers to investigate the conditions that need to be in place to encourage people to comply with social distancing rules or to adopt specific personal protective behaviour. People might, for example, be willing to use hand sanitiser regularly, especially if they feel that this is the right thing to do (behaviour-related *attitude*) and think that it will benefit them and others (behaviour-related *belief*). Their motivation to do this might get even stronger if they think that other people are doing this and that they should therefore conform as well (*subjective norm*). In the end, though, they might find it difficult to use hand sanitiser regularly if they cannot find any and cannot afford to buy their own (*behavioural control*).

Hence, understanding the nature of all these elements and how they stack up together in mutually supportive ways (or not) can provide valuable insights into communications that might be devised and other steps that might be taken to ensure that a specific behaviour can and does take place.

Reframing Compliance within a Rational Model of Behavioural Control

It is worth pausing to reflect on the answers behavioural modelling might provide in terms of whether continued public commitment to restrictions on their everyday behaviour was near to failing. The theory of planned behaviour identified a number of internal psychological factors that could either promote or impede behaviour change. Evidence emerged internationally during the 2020 pandemic, in which behavioural compliance was examined within the framework of this theoretical model. It might then be useful to revisit some polling evidence from within the United Kingdom to detect whether these internal factors were in a state to strengthen or weaken behavioural compliance.

A mainstay of lockdowns used in many countries was "social distancing". The principal manifestations of this intervention in terms of human behaviour were that people limited their physical contact with others from outside their household; they maintained a one- to two-metre distance between themselves and others when they did meet; they avoided travelling far from home; and they only left home occasionally for essential reasons. While most people, across many countries, complied with these restrictions, they did place a strain on the lives of many. Not everyone complied fully all the time and certainly as time went by and populations were confronted with repeat lockdowns after periods of restriction relaxation, more compliance breaches occurred.

In learning lessons for the future, we need to know what were the forces that really drove behavioural compliance during pandemic lockdowns and other periods of lighter touch restrictions. We might speculate that people kept themselves locked away because they were afraid or out of a sense of civic duty, but does this provide a comprehensive explanation of what was going on?

An international study of adherence to behavioural measures to fight back against the spread of COVID-19 surveyed people from eight countries: France, Germany, Poland, Russia, Spain, Sweden, the United Kingdom and the United States (Margraf et al., 2020). Well over 7,000 people took part. Across the whole sample, three-quarters of respondents (74%) rated their government's interventions as "useful" and over nine in ten (92%) said they adhered to them. There were some variances between countries. Adherence was lowest in Poland and Russia, where people felt abandoned by their governments. It was also low in Sweden and the United States, where there had been some initial ambivalence towards imposing severe restrictions on people's behaviour. The most compliant populations were found in France, Germany, Spain and the United Kingdom.

Compliance was predicted by being female, older, from a higher-risk heath group, being affected physically and mentally by the restrictions, having greater trust in government information, and feeling better informed. The theory of planned behaviour was utilised to interpret the findings. Evidence emerged that having more positive attitudes towards and beliefs about behavioural restrictions were important to behaviour change along with the perception that others were being compliant and the feeling that support was being offered to make the restrictions more doable. Together, these internal psychological processes predicted a higher probability of compliance with restrictions (Margraf et al., 2020).

Another study investigated compliance with an international sample of respondents recruited across Europe and North America within this theoretical model (Coroiu et al., 2020). Respondents were asked to endorse various possible reasons as to why they observed social distancing restrictions on their own behaviour. An overwhelming sense of civic responsibility emerged from some findings, with more than eight in ten respondents saying they engaged in social distancing because they wanted to protect others (85%) as much as themselves (84%) and also that they felt a responsibility to protect their community (84%).

In exploring potential barriers to compliance, the research revealed that a large minority of respondents observed that there were many people walking in the streets around where they lived, and therefore inferring that many people seemed not to be following the restrictions to the latter (31%). In addition, from their own perspective, they had family members or friends for whom they ran errands because they were not able to do certain things for themselves (25%). This last point illustrated the inner tensions with which people had to wrestle when balancing their own behavioural compliance with a need to demonstrate a different kind of duty towards loved ones and close friends who needed their help. Another barrier noted only by a few (13%) was that they did not always trust the messages produced about the pandemic by their own government. The same proportion also said they themselves often felt stressed when they spent a lot of time alone (13%). This feeling no doubt gave rise to temptations to seek out the company of others despite being told this was the wrong thing to do. In general, however, virtually everybody (90%) said they avoided crowded places and non-essential travel (Coroiu et al., 2020).

Social distancing as an intervention can prove to be effective in controlling the spread of the novel coronavirus, but this result is dependent on people's compliance with the rules surrounding it. Research into what makes people comply with rules which restrict their normal behaviour has shown that public behaviour could be influenced by perceptions of government policies and actions. One study of people living in Kuwait, South Korea and the United States showed that positive public opinion about the attempts being made by their government to control the spread of the new virus and protect the population strengthened people's willingness to comply with social distancing restrictions. The perception also that government was motivated, in its policies and action, to create a setting in which it would be safe to re-open businesses also seemed to motivate people to play their part through social distancing. Those people that sought out more information related to the pandemic, including via social media, tended also to report a stronger willingness to comply with restrictions on their normal behaviour (Al-Hasan et al., 2020).

Perceived threat and ability to cope with the pandemic are important reactions among members of the public because these mental states will also shape people's behaviour. In a study of people in the United States, Kuwait and South Korea, it was found that perceived threat from COVID-19 was greater among those who sought out more information about it from various source, and especially from social media. Greater perceived threat from COVID-19 and a stronger perceived ability to cope with it were also positively related to propensity to adhere to social distancing rules. Paying more attention to relevant information sources also improved people's knowledge about what was going on and this also strengthened their willingness to comply with social distancing restrictions. These effects were significant in all the countries investigated, but were strongest in the United States (Al-Hasan et al., 2020).

In the Philippines, the country was placed under quarantine for six months from 17th March 2020. Yet, on the 16th July 2020, the country was declared to have the highest number of COVID-19 cases (61,266 and 1,643 deaths). The so-called "enhanced community quarantine" imposed in Luzon by the Philippines government was the longest total lockdown in the world. Research was conducted to find out more about how people responded, behaviourally, to the government's restrictions on their activities. The researchers surveyed 649 Filipinos about COVID-19, their vulnerability, their government's use of different intervention measures, their intention to follow these measures and their views about their effectiveness (Prasetyo et al., 2020).

Two theories, Protection Motivation Theory (PMT) and the Theory of Planned Behaviour, were adopted to examine causal relationships between people's behavioural compliance and the perceived effectiveness of the restrictions. With PMT, when individuals are confronted with a threatening event, they are motivated to adopt some form of protective behaviour if they can. The prevailing belief in this context is that by taking preventative steps further threats can be abated, whereas inaction means that continue to be a problem. Being prepared for a threat can help to alleviate it and preparation generally means developing an understanding about it and the types of risks it represents. In theory, the greater our understanding of a threat, such as a new and highly infectious virus, the more we can get its perceived severity in perspective and also the less personally vulnerable to it we feel. The theory of planned behaviour meanwhile predicted that behaviour change or adoption is underpinned by attitudes towards the behaviour, perceptions of the behavioural norms of the community and finally by a perception that the behaviour itself is feasible or within the grasp of the individual.

Another concept that is relevant to the theory of planned behaviour and protection motivation theory is "self-efficacy". This is closely linked to "perceived behavioural control" and concerns the skillsets a person has that are relevant to their response or decision making in any specific situation (Bandura, 1977, 1978). This factor will come into play in settings, such as the pandemic, where people are requested to make changes to their normal behaviour patterns and/or to adopt new specific behaviours, for example, in the context of protecting themselves from an external risk (Workman et al., 2008).

The concept of "subjective norm" is defined in terms of the group or community-wide needs that specific action can cater to and the benefits or rewards that follow from it and, most importantly, the extent to which these functions and outcomes are widely recognised by others in an individual's community or the wider population. If individuals are requested to change their normal behaviour and to adopt specific new behaviours, they will be more likely to comply if they can witness others around them doing the same. This propensity is strengthened still further when those "others" represent important social reference points or role models for individuals. Even if they have not seen such role models directly, if they receive information from a credible and trusted source that clearly indicates that the requested behaviour is being widely adopted or that there is a general expectation "among people" that it should be, then their probability of following suit increases (Grimes & Marquardson, 2019; Ho et al., 2017).

While subjective norms can mediate intentions to behave as requested, they might come up against other persuasive influences that counter their effects.

One example of this influence might be alternative worldviews about the behaviour being requested other than that which currently underpins it (Armitage & Conner, 2001). Hence, we might be told by authorities that getting vaccinated against COVID-19 is the eventual solution to the problem only then to be confronted with alternative messages questioning whether vaccines are safe.

The attitude that people have towards a requested change to behaviour tends to be defined by whether an internalised orientation develops towards the behaviour that qualifies whether it is a good thing or a bad thing to do. This perception can be influenced by personal behavioural experiences and also by information about it received from others. In the case of COVID-19, compliance with restrictive behaviour rules might be classed as a good thing both because it will serve to protect the individual and also because it will help to end the pandemic quickly and this will be best for the greater good. Holding a positive disposition towards a behaviour has been found historically to enhance the likelihood that it will be adopted (McMillan & Conner, 2003; Sasse et al., 2002). A negative attitude towards the behaviour, regardless of its rationale, will generally weaken the likelihood of compliance (Myyry et al., 2009; Pahnila et al., 2007).

If internal beliefs and perceptions are lined up in the appropriate way, they will individually and collectively increase a person's intention (or motivation) to perform a desired behaviour. The presence of this intention will then reinforce the likelihood that the behaviour will be executed (Mahardika et al., 2020).

In the Philippines research, the public's perception of the disease risk was influenced by their understanding of its severity and their own vulnerability. This understanding also includes awareness of which groups in society were at most risk from the disease. Of the three planned behaviour variables, attitudes, subjective norms and perceived behavioural control together, understanding about the virus was related to subjective norm beliefs and perceived behavioural control (Prasetyo et al., 2020).

One interpretation of the first of these relationships was that understanding about the virus and how to avoid catching it may have been influenced by seeing other people in the community observing preventive protocols such as staying home, maintaining a physical distance from others and wearing face masks when mingling with other people outside the home. Stronger perceptions of personal vulnerability were related to weaker behavioural control beliefs. When surrounded by people following the rules, perceived vulnerability is lessened and feelings of being able to control one's own fate get stronger. These factors would also be expected to impact on attitude towards the virus and preventive behaviour to cope with it (Armitage & Conner, 2001).

Together attitude towards the virus and preventive or protection behaviour, subjective norm perceptions and perception of being able to take behavioural control of the situation strengthened individuals' intentions to comply with protective measures introduced by the government. This intention to follow the rules was in turn related to actual behavioural compliance, or at least as it was reported by these Filipino respondents. Actual behaviour here represented compliance with the rules such as wearing a face mask or observing physical distancing rules. In addition, another variable, called adaptive behaviour, measured behaviour changes adopted by the individual during the pandemic, such as trying to eat healthy and trying to work from home as much as possible. Both adaptive behaviour and more direct compliance behaviour were more likely among those people with the right COVID protection attitudes, subjective norm perceptions and behavioural control beliefs. Finally, the perceived effectiveness of these protective behaviours was stronger among those performing these behaviours (Prasetyo et al., 2020).

Theory of Planned Behaviour and Compliance with COVID-19 Restrictions

Although regular and explicit environmental reminders about behaviour change or subtle signals that nudge people unwittingly in a specific behavioural direction can be effective to producing behaviour change outcomes, sometimes they are not enough and will only work effectively under specific conditions. Sometimes, the drive to change behaviour must come from within and not simply from external stimuli. People must make rational judgements about specific courses of action based on their thoughts and feelings about these actions and their perceptions of what other people are doing and of what might be behaviourally possible for them.

The theory of planned behaviour has been used as a model to test the efficacy of COVID-19 restrictions designed to control the spread of the new coronavirus. Research using this model was conducted in different parts of the world with samples drawn from the public and a number of professional groups. This model was designed to investigate the mediating effects of people's beliefs and attitudes associated with the behaviour they were being encouraged to adopt or change, the extent to which they perceive that other people had endorsed or were also compliant with this behaviour (normative beliefs), and the extent to which those being investigated believed they would be able to change their behaviour (control beliefs).

Social distancing was introduced around the world as a primary non-pharmaceutical intervention (NPI) with which to control the spread of the new coronavirus. This intervention could only work if most people complied with it. Many polls indicated widespread self-reported compliance, but the extent of this could vary between different self-protective personal hygiene and social distancing behaviours.

There is much past research to show that these internal psychological variables can work so as to increase the strength of specific behavioural intentions and likelihood of the behaviour itself making an appearance (McEachan et al., 2011). This model has been used to influence alcohol consumption, food choices, use of condoms or of sunscreens and adoption of specific treatments for serious illness (Andrew et al., 2016; Cooke et al., 2016; McDermott et al., 2015; Rich et al., 2015; Starfelt Sutton & White, 2016).

A number of studies demonstrated that the theory of planned behaviour model could be used to predict compliance with COVID-19 prevention behaviours (Das et al., 2020). Other studies have used extended versions of the original model to achieve the same results (Ahmad et al., 2020; Callow et al., 2020). In a study of people in Bangladesh, positive attitudes towards social distancing, perceptions of social pressures to conform to this behaviour and perceived competence to do so all predicted intentions to comply in the future (Das et al., 2020).

One of the earliest outbreaks of COVID-19 in Europe occurred in Italy. The country went into lockdown between 9th March and 18th May 2020. People were told to stay at home as much as possible. By 4th May, people had the freedom to see relatives and from 18th May, they were allowed to see their friends, but still had to observe strict social distancing rules. An Italian study of just over 400 people assessed predictors of hand hygiene and social distancing compliance using the theory of planned behaviour (Trifiletti et al., 2021).

Having more positive attitudes towards these behaviours, belief in their efficacy, the perception that others were being compliant and the belief among respondents that they would be able to comply predicted compliance with these behaviours when socialising with others. Risk perceptions were measured as well and were found to make no difference to propensity to wash hands regularly but had a statistically significant but rather weak relationship to social distancing compliance. Other evidence emerged to show that risk perceptions were weak predictors of adoption of preventive behaviours (Clark et al., 2020).

The feeling of having control over one's own behaviour is important in the context of taking personal steps to prevent or protect oneself from a threat to health. This factor can be especially important when people feel more generally constrained in how they may behave. Under circumstances, where surrounding social conditions are defined by uncertainty, individuals seek convenient and available ways of taking whatever control they can. Any advice which points them in the right direction in this context is likely to have an impact. While internalised attitudes and beliefs concerning a behaviour or object and perceived social norms relating to it can work together to increase an intention to change or adopt a specific behaviour, actually following through ultimately depends upon whether the individual feels able to perform that behaviour (Ajzen, 1991; Armitage & Conner, 2001; Kiriakidis, 2015).

The internalised attitudes and beliefs about a behaviour together with "subjective norms" can therefore prove to be effective in predicting behavioural intention but not actual behaviour. Very often, some experts have argued, people misjudge just how capable they might be in respect of embracing a behaviour change (Sheeran et al., 2003).

A UK survey of students examined their perceptions of the effectiveness of protective measures against COVID-19 and relationships of other perceptions and beliefs on their intentions to follow these protective measures themselves (Barrett & Cheung, 2021). The principal protective measures under consideration here were social distancing and hand hygiene. This research was undertaken in May 2020 during the country's first lockdown. Most students displayed good knowledge about the effectiveness of these interventions. The propensity to follow such practices was predicted by students' perceptions of their efficacy; the advantages and benefits accrued from such behaviour and trust in the policy underpinning it. The latter measures represented the internal attitude and belief towards changed behaviour components of the theory of planned behaviour.

Perceived discrimination based on perceptions that other people had discriminated against them because of their presumed COVID-19 status was negatively associated with intended future social distancing compliance. Such perceived discrimination weakens perceptions of personal control over future health behaviour and therefore discourage people from complying fully with public health restrictions on their everyday behaviour.

A much bigger study of adherence to behavioural measures to fight back against the spread of COVID-19 surveyed people from eight countries: France, Germany, Poland, Russia, Spain, Sweden, the United Kingdom and the United States (Margraf et al., 2020). Well over 7,000 people took part. Across the whole sample, three-quarters of respondents (74%) rated their government's interventions as "useful" and over nine in ten (92%) said they adhered to them. There were some variances between countries. Adherence was lowest in Poland and Russia, where people felt abandoned by their governments. It was also low in Sweden and the United States, where there had been some initial ambivalence towards imposing severe restrictions on people's behaviour. The most compliant populations were found in France, Germany, Spain and the United Kingdom.

Compliance was predicted by being female, older, from a higher-risk heath group, being affected physically and mentally by the restrictions, having greater trust in government information, and feeling better informed. The theory of planned behaviour was utilised to interpret the findings. Evidence emerged that having more positive attitudes towards and beliefs about behavioural restrictions, the perception that others were being compliant and the feeling that support was being offered to make the restrictions more doable predicted a higher probability of compliance with restrictions.

Research showed that the theory of planned behaviour model was able to predict the likelihood that students would wear face masks in the context of a fictional future pandemic (Chan et al., 2015). In another study that studied people's behaviour choices in a real pandemic, the theory of planned behaviour (TPB) predicted people's willingness to engage in self-protective behaviours during the 2003 severe acute respiratory syndrome (SARS) outbreak (Cheng & Ng, 2006). This study grouped various protective behaviours together and failed to separate out the likelihood that each on would be adopted. The researchers lumped together 15 different behaviours that represented a variety of actions including handwashing, disinfecting surfaces, socially isolating, gathering more relevant information, and trying to improve general state of health. It cannot be assumed that each of these behaviours was likely to change to same degree.

In another study in China, the TPB was able to predict the probability that parents with children under the age of 18 along with factory workers were likely to get vaccinated (Zhang et al., 2020, 2021). Elsewhere, it was found that having a positive attitude towards adoption of interventions to tackle an epidemic increased motivation to adopt preventive behaviours, but perception of what other people might do was not related to this behaviour outcome. Ultimately, whether individuals felt able to make the necessary behaviour changes (perceived behaviour control) was critical and could undermine the likelihood of target behaviour being adopted all by itself (Ahmad et al., 2020).

Focus group research with a small sample of UK adults found that some claimed to be committed adherents to social distancing guidelines and were aware of non-adherence in others, but this did not weaken their own resolve. Some people also displayed lingering uncertainty about risks going forward once restrictions were lifted despite many wanting life to return to normal. Then there were individuals who felt extreme loss of meaning of life and self-worth because of social isolation and for some of these individuals it was clear there might be perceived behaviour control problems in terms of their longer-term compliance with COVID-19 regulations. Then, there were participants who found a lack of clarity in the guidelines and a loss of trust in government and its messaging. These negative attitudes undermined their willingness to comply with government guidelines (Williams et al., 2020).

These findings were derived from open-ended interviews and cannot provide the kinds of data needed to demonstrate causal relationships between internal psychological states and subsequent behaviour. Nonetheless, the research offered some insights into people's thought processes about the pandemic and the restrictions being deployed by the government. Potential psychological barriers to compliance could be identified for further investigation in modelling studies, which were better equipped to understand how public behaviour could be effectively controlled.

In a different approach to the study of public compliance with pandemic restrictions, one group of researchers collected data via social media sites such as Facebook, NextDoor and Twitter. Participants could respond openly in free text form. There were no multiple-choice questions to constrain their responses. Computerised natural language analysis tools were used to analyse the large amounts of text produced. In just nine days, the researchers had amassed over 20,000 responses, although not everyone who replied in total had responded to every question. Participants were asked to provide their age so that comparisons could be made of the responses of different age groups (Moore et al., 2020).

Younger people were emotionally more negative about the pandemic and its restrictions on public behaviour. They displayed more self-centred opinions about the pros and cons of lockdowns and were less concerned about risks to their family than the collateral impact of constraints on their own activities. Older people were more concerned about their families, but they were also concerned for themselves if they were in a higher risk category. Yet, older people were not an anxious as might have been expected given their sensitivity to COVID-19 risks.

The youngest adults (aged 18–31) had the lowest reported compliance rates with COVID-19 restrictions. They were anxious and this anxiety appeared also to drive their behaviour. In the context of a model such as the theory of planned behaviour, young people were concerned about the mental health impact of being starved of normal social contact and also believed it was important to get back to normal activities as early as possible, not least work-related activities. Some also believed that the authorities had over-reacted and that a general lockdown was overkill in terms of the measures they believed would be sufficient to slow the spread of the disease. The researchers believed that public health messages need to focus more on young people because they were likely to be the most resistant to behavioural compliance, especially if they felt unable to comply because of a lack of belief in the restrictions and the pain of side effects.

The Predictive Strength of Theory of Planned Behaviour Constructs

Evidence has emerged during the COVID-19 pandemic that perceived behaviour control and self-efficacy were linked to behaviour intentions and overt behaviour. These variables were found to be significant predictors of social distancing behaviour, personal hygiene and staying home when symptomatic (Lin et al., 2020). In another study, subjective norms and perceived behaviour control emerged as the best predictors of intentions to wash hands, avoid face touching, stay home when sick, cover nose and mouth when coughing or sneezing and use a face mask (Andarge et al., 2020).

Yu et al. (2021) reported that positive (but not negative) attitudes towards a behaviour, subjective norms and perceived behavioural control combined to motivate social distancing behaviour in China. Belief in the effectiveness of the behaviour was found to be sufficient in another study to motivate use of hand sanitiser and avoidance of gatherings of people outside one's home (Pan et al., 2020).

An online survey of 10,000 people in China questioned them about their use of Chinese traditional medicines during the COVID-19 outbreak. Many people in China believed that these ancient medicines could strengthen the body's resistance to all kinds of diseases. Questions probed respondents' positive or negative feelings about this behaviour, their perceptions of the normality of the behaviour among others in their community and the ease or difficulty with which they could engage in the behaviour. It was hypothesised, according to the theory of planned behaviour, that if all these internal psychological components could be lined up in the same way, they would create conditions in which increased motivation to turn to alternative medicines would result. The data confirmed these hypotheses. Past behaviour also emerged as a critical variable that determined more than anything else whether the behaviour being predicted would take place again (Xia et al., 2021).

Research from Hong Kong measured public compliance with three types of social distancing behaviours: number of close physical contacts in a day in public venues, the frequencies of avoiding social gatherings and the levels of physical distancing in public venues. When respondents were surveyed in April 2020, they were found on average to report just over 15 close physical contacts per day in public spaces. Around eight in ten said they avoided social gatherings. Only just over one in three (35%) said they avoided public transport. Positive attitudes towards these behaviours (that is not seeing them as inconvenient and also as necessary), together with subjective norms (i.e., perceptions that other people were compliant and expected it) and perceived behavioural control (i.e., acknowledging that these behaviours were within their personal efficacy) all motivated compliance (Yu et al., 2021).

An Australian study used an extended version of the theory of planned behaviour alongside measures of participants' knowledge and understanding of social distancing measures as predictors of intentions to adhere to behavioural restrictions (Sturman et al., 2021). Participants were recruited in Melbourne during a period of heightened social distancing restrictions. Melbourne experienced a number of general lockdowns including one that lasted for over 100 days. The researchers constructed vignettes to assess participants' willingness to comply with restrictions. A willingness to comply with social distancing rules was predicted statistically by having positive attitudes towards the restrictions and these were in turn linked to knowledge about the restrictions. A perceived ability to adhere to restrictions (i.e., perceived behavioural control) was also another factor that was related to motivation to comply.

An online survey of more than 3,000 adults in Quebec, Canada, conducted in June 2020, measured COVID-19 related perceptions and fears, adherence to social distancing rules and perceptions of subjective norms linked to social distancing and respondents' perceived behavioural control over such behaviour and how all these factors were related to intentions to comply with social distancing rules in the future. Perceptions of risks associated with COVID-19 and fears about infection had some bearing on intentions to keep a minimum physical distance from others, but the theory of planned behaviour constructs, subjective norms and perceived behavioural control, were also strongly linked to these behavioural intentions and further strengthened the effects of risk perceptions and fears. Hence, internalised beliefs about COVID-19 and about behavioural interventions were important to intentions to comply with behaviour restrictions, but beliefs about how other people were behaving and about own ability to comply were key predictors (Frounfelker et al., 2021).

In the United States, a longitudinal survey of respondents from 48 states collected data at baseline and then three months later during the pandemic. The research was theoretically underpinned by the theory of planned behaviour. The main focus was on explaining people's willingness and intentions to comply with social distancing rules. Evidence emerged positive attitudes towards social distancing strengthened over time, but subjective norms (i.e., perceptions that other people were being compliant) weakened and perceived behaviour control (or assessed ability to be able to comply) remained stable. All three of these variables were significantly related to baseline intentions to be compliant with social distancing rules. Yet, over time, compliance was found to grow weaker, although those with stronger intentions around social distancing in the first survey also displayed the strongest intentions to continue to do so at the second wave (Gibson et al., 2021). This research shows that if people are appropriately motivated early in a pandemic to comply with behavioural restrictions, they will remain this way in the future. Over time, however, both the motivated and non-motivated will display weaker intentions to comply with restrictions to their behaviour.

A cross-national survey conducted in Australia and the United States used theory of planned behaviour constructs (attitude, subjective norm, perceived behavioural control) and measured behavioural intentions, action planning and past habits and behaviour with respect to social distancing behaviour at two time points one week apart (Hagger et al., 2020). Subjective norm and perceived behaviour control emerged as significant predictors of social distancing intentions. Reported past behaviour was also an important predictor of future intentions but this did not dilute the significance of perceived social norms and self-efficacy in terms of own behaviour. Once again, all theory of planned behaviour constructs was found to have value in predicting people's future behaviour intentions in relation to the pandemic.

Another study investigated predictors of intentions to perform eight different preventive behaviours: washing hands, using hand sanitiser, not touching your face, social distancing, wearing a face mask, disinfecting surfaces, coughing in your elbow and staying home if sick (Aschwanden et al., 2021). Over 2,200 people were surveyed about these behaviours in the United States, aged between 18 and 98. Further measures were taken of theory of planned behaviour constructs, including attitudes towards preventive behaviours, perceptions of norms of behaviour among others, and perceived behavioural control.

Perceived behavioural control was measured as follows. "To reduce the spread of the coronavirus, how DIFFICULT is it for you to follow these recommendations?" Response options were extremely easy, somewhat easy, neither easy nor difficult, somewhat difficult and extremely difficult. Perceived subjective norm asked respondents: "To reduce the spread of the coronavirus, how many OTHER PEOPLE do you think are following these recommendations?" Response options were: no one, few people, some people, most people, everyone. Attitude towards each preventive behaviour was measured by asking respondents: "To reduce the spread of the coronavirus, how EFFECTIVE do you believe these recommendations are?" Responses ranged on a five-point scale from extremely effective to extremely ineffective.

Each of the theory of planned behaviour variables was found to have independent associations with each preventive behaviour. Perceived behavioural control emerged across most preventive behaviours as the variable most strongly linked to preventive behaviour intentions, especially for older adults. There were some variances in findings. Subjective norm was not associated significantly with intention to comply with "coughing into your elbow". Attitude towards the behaviour was more strongly related to social distancing intention than was perceived behaviour control or subjective norm.

Theory of Planned Behaviour and Behaviour Change among Health Professionals

Research within the theory of planned behaviour framework was conducted with one group of clinical professionals – dentists – to find out whether it could provide insights into ways of motivating COVID-compliance with professional practice. This investigation was conducted with 324 dental health-care workers in Saudi Arabia. Respondents' intentions to comply with relevant COVID-19 restrictions designed to control spread of infections were underpinned to some degree by having positive attitudes about whether this would be a good thing to do (Shubayr et al., 2020).

A number of dentists, dental hygienists and their assistants were surveyed online about the infection protection practices used in their profession. Respondents' knowledge of these practices was tested together with their beliefs in their efficacy. For example: "Practicing COVID-19 IPC will protect the staff in the dental clinic". Attitudes towards these practices were measured with questions that invited respondents to react positively or negatively towards their use. A list of statements concerning the protection of staff and others in their dental clinic was rated in terms of their importance.

The perception that others, especially relevant others, would also be compliant represented a further motivation of intention of respondents to be compliant themselves. A typical statement was: "Most colleagues who are important to me practice COVID-19 IPC regularly in their dental clinic".

Perceived behaviour control was measured through a further series of statements, such as: "I am confident that I have enough experience to practice COVID-19 IPC on a regular basis in my clinic", and "I have enough time and resources to practice COVID-19 IPC on a regular basis in my clinic".

Multivariate analyses showed that attitudes towards COVID interventions and the perceptions that other colleagues were compliant (i.e., subjective norms) were significantly predictive of intentions to be behaviourally compliant and explained 44% of the variance in compliance. Other moderating variables from this model such as general beliefs about the efficacy of the interventions or respondents' perceptions of their ability to comply were not significant predictors of intention to comply (Shubayr et al., 2020).

Dental academics across 28 countries completed a questionnaire online about their stress levels, fears and worries about COVID-19; subjective perceptions on threat were based on national COVID fatality data and their perceived ability to control the situation through their professional training. They were then also asked about their own use of protective behaviours such as regular handwashing and avoidance of crowded spaces.

More frequent handwashing and avoidance of crowded places were predicted by exhibiting greater stress, which was in turn influenced by their own fears of infection, worries because of their own profession and worries because of restricted mobility. Low national fatality rates were associated with more frequent handwashing and avoidance of crowded places. The findings showed that health professionals could experience considerable stress because of COVID-19 and no matter how well trained they had been, especially in dealing with public emergencies, this reaction did not change. In keeping with predictions that would be made by the theory of planned behaviour, their own protective behaviours did not just boil down to their professional training, but were also influenced by their own COVID-related attitudes, subjective norm perceptions and ability to believe they were able to take action to protect themselves (Ammar et al., 2020).

A study with 556 Romanians and 181 Kazakhs examined the impact of exposure to information about COVID-19 on people's attitudes and beliefs about the new virus and the likelihood in turn that they would adopt protective behavioural measures against infection by it (Curseu et al., 2021).

The researchers found that exposure to information about the new coronavirus promoted negative attitudes towards it and also subjective norms relating to the steps that people were taking against it. These effects were diluted, however, when relevant informational messaging contained humour. This is not a factor that the theory of planned behaviour would usually have taken into account and indicates why some behavioural scientists have offered an extended model, as we will see in the next chapter.

In line with the predictions of the theory of planned behaviour, elsewhere it was reported that if information about COVID-19 promoted the right attitudes about the disease and about protective behaviour that can be used against it, drew attention to the wider concerns and willingness to take action among the wider community and left individuals believing it was within their capabilities to do something about it, then intentions to adopt recommended protective behaviours also emerged. Stronger negative attitudes towards COVID-19 in particular predicted increased probability of adoption of protective behaviours. Despite the stronger negative attitudes of older people than young people, there were no age differences in motivation to take protective steps. Furthermore, negative feelings about COVID-19 could also strengthen over time, but this did not invariably translate into progressively greater likelihood of taking protective steps (Curseu et al., 2021).

Without Behaviour Control, Behaviour Change Is Less Likely

Judgements about whether adopting a specific pattern of behaviour is feasible even when an individual recognises there are good personal or societal reasons for doing so will be affected by perceived difficulties that pertain to that person's own situation. Citizens might be prepared to accept the need to behave in a responsible way when their country faces a national crisis such as with the COVID-19 pandemic. When restrictive behaviours, designed to halt the spread of the disease, require people to put themselves at other considerable risks, their motivation to do "the right thing" can become severely tested.

The theory of planned behaviour causes us to take into account the significant impact on any final behavioural impact of a persuasive behaviour change campaign or "perceived behavioural control". Even when internalised beliefs and attitudes associated with that target behaviour change outcome stack up in its favour, eventual behaviour change might be rejected or only partially accepted and adopted when the harm it could cause is regarded as more serious than any it might protect against. One of the biggest barriers to behaviour change in the pandemic was the economic and financial harm caused to individuals by staying off work or being laid off temporarily while the employer they worked for closed their business.

Evidence from the United States demonstrated that factors such as job security and financial insecurity could be critical to the success of behaviour change programmes during the COVID-19 pandemic. In one study, data were collected from a sample of over 700 workers covering 43 states (Probst et al., 2020). In states with restrictive pandemic intervention policies, it was the people with the greatest financial security who were most likely to report their compliance with these interventions. Those who were less financially secure or, more accurately, who were financially insecure, were far less likely to do so. Hence, while some might argue that more restrictive behavioural measures (e.g., more extensive and vigilant application of socially distancing rules) provided greater protection to the public, these interventions provided greater benefit for the financially secure who could afford to adopt them.

It could be argued that this finding was an empirical discovery during the pandemic and that this type of "behaviour control" barrier to public compliance was demonstrated but may not have been known in advance. This is the "hindsight" defence. In fact, social scientists had developed an explanation of this phenomenon based of "scarcity theory" some years earlier. This theory recognised that when people perceive future (or current) shortages of essential commodities or resources, their behaviour focuses on finding immediate solutions. This mindset can take priority over all others (Mani et al., 2013; Mullainathan & Shafir, 2014). Once individuals enter this type of cognitive state, they lack the capacity mentally to tune into other behavioural demands (Huijsmans et al., 2019; Shah et al., 2012).

People's concerns about critical aspects of their own and their families' survival occupy their attention fully and leave no room psychologically for any other considerations. When behaviour change requests are made of them that can be accommodated alongside these concerns, there may be some adoption of those behaviours. In the context of the pandemic, however, personal hygiene safety recommendations such as regular handwashing and sanitisation and washing down of surfaces could, for some with financial insecurity, represent additional costs they cannot afford. Similarly, social distancing requirements might also be difficult to embrace where they resulted in loss of income.

Further research has shed light on the psychological processes that could impact upon the ability to comply with behaviour restrictions. When people suffer negative shocks, these experiences can change their cognitive functioning in that moment and beyond. Such shocks might involve threats to people's employment, their physical health, their mental health or involve other forms of stressful event. When they have had these experiences, they might for a time perform less effectively when making other decisions. They might also be more prone to blame others for things that are going wrong in their own lives.

In a cognitive context, negative stressors can impede judgement, that is, the ability to filter out extraneous distraction to be able to focus fully on matters requiring their immediate attention, and could disrupt their abilities to store and remember new information (Baddeley & Hitch, 2020; Diamond, 2013). Under these conditions, many individuals become more risk averse and are less likely to forfeit a benefit today for a better benefit that will come later (Arrow, 1971; Pratt, 1964).

It is not difficult to see how being in this cognitive state might impede people's willingness to adopt restrictions to their normal behaviours when such restrictions pose immediate threats that are themselves highly stressful and when the "reward" of performing a public good that will deliver a significant beneficial later (i.e., protection of self and others from a highly infectious and airborne virus) is an outcome they will not or cannot recognise (Bowles & Polanía-Reyes, 2012).

When individuals become focused on themselves because there are stressors present in their environment that represent a real personal threat, they are less likely to prefer behaviour change requests that are seen to offer no relevant personal protection or offers only a kind of protection that is outweighed by the harms caused by compliance with these requests.

These effects were demonstrated in a survey conducted over two waves one week apart with samples in Spain and the United Kingdom during the first lockdowns in April 2020 (Bogliacino et al., 2021). Respondents were tested on their judgements about risks, willingness to sacrifice a freedom or benefit today for a better one tomorrow (also called "time preference"), altruistic tendencies, trust in others and other preferences. They were also randomly split into two sub-samples. One group was asked to recall a negative and stressful event from their lives and the other group recalled a neutral or positive life event. The two sub-samples were then compared on their responses to the judgements outlined earlier. They were also given a cognitive performance test to test their general cognitive abilities. The researchers also classified the stressful life events as those linked to economic and job security, physical or mental health issues or other stressful events.

Their findings showed that those recalling a negative shock event performed more poorly than did those recalling a neutral or positive event on general cognitive performance tasks and they were also the more risk averse of the two sub-samples. The researchers believed these differences in performance could be explained more by cognitive capacity effects than emotional impact effects. In other words, it is not that when people remembered a negative life event, the emotional reaction this might have interfered with the abilities to make sound judgements and solve probes. These response outcomes were, they believed, more likely to drive from the way in which cognitive processing capacity was directed by stressors. Cognitive functioning could become more narrowly focused on the stressor and how to resolve it leaving much reduced capacity for making other judgements. Hence, in terms of behavioural control, the failure to take control to change behaviour in a desired fashion is determined not just by social and economic consideration but also by effective cognitive processing of relevant information that feeds into control decision making.

Concluding Observations

Social distancing measures require the voluntary compliance of populations. As an intervention it brings costs with it. People are then placed in a position where they must weigh up the costs and benefits of social distancing. There would be individuals for whom the costs of social distancing outweigh the benefits and then compliance with behavioural restrictions can present a difficult challenge. As previously reviewed evidence indicated, very often, the costs of social distancing were economic. Taking time off work or being laid off for an indefinite period meant loss of income. This could represent an intolerable stressor for many households with low incomes. To persuade people to change their behaviour in ways that could cause such problems and potential personal damage to control something novel or unknown that could have even worse effects will always be a challenge. People must believe that the cause is just and that it will be effective. They must weigh up the costs and benefits of compliance and non-compliance with behaviour change demands of authorities. They must also decide whether they trust these authorities to give the right advice for the right reasons.

What has become apparent as well is that being placed in a situation such as lockdown with social distancing rules that meant little interaction with others could create stresses for many people that could also interfere with their ability to make sound and considered judgements about their behaviour. When people's core cognitive capacities are overburdened with concerns about being able to get essential resources for themselves and their families, they have significantly reduced capacity to take note of constantly changing rules and regulations concerning public behaviour (Xie et al., 2020).

Social distancing rules can be effective in slowing or stopping the spread of infectious airborne viruses but only if people comply with them. With social distancing rules that remain largely voluntary, high rates of non-compliance could be expected where the costs of compliance, at least in the short-term, were perceived to outweigh their benefits. When people are placed in this kind of situation, they will tend to give higher priority to costs than to benefits (Reluga, 2010). This inclination renders the goal of widespread public behaviour control even more of a challenge.

One important facet of the cognitive issue raised by stressors is the impact that they have on "working memory". This is the part of memory where new and incoming information is sifted and interpreted with relevant knowledge from long-term memory stores being referenced at the same time. The working memory has a limited processing capacity. Where lots of different inputs are received within a short period of time, those that stand out the most will command the greatest attention and be most likely to make it into longer-term storage (Cowan, 2001; Luck & Vogel, 2013; Zhang & Luck, 2013).

Individuals with greater working memory capacity might be better placed to process and remember social distancing rules. They will then be better placed to follow those rules. If they are under stress, however, this processing could be undermined. Effective processing of social distancing rules would then enable people to conduct their own cost-benefit analysis of the impact of compliance with these restrictions on their behaviour. The less people comply with social distancing rules, of course, the less effective it will be as an intervention in a pandemic. Early non-compliance might be explained in part by the initial stress many people felt when lockdown restrictions were introduced. The restrictions on their everyday behaviour could have had significant impact on them economically and psychologically. Such stress might then had disrupted their working memory at a time when they needed to pay attention to new rules of public behaviour.

Research in the United States confirmed that those people with greater working memory capacity did also exhibit greater social distancing compliance. The researchers surveyed a national sample of Americans distributed across different states during March 2020 when the US lockdowns had just begun. Respondents were given a simple working memory test and also asked to self-report on their social distancing compliance. The relationship between working memory capacity and social distancing compliance survived controls for gender, age, education, socioeconomic status, intelligence and personality (Xie et al., 2020).

Put another way, there appears to be a specific characteristic linked to a person's established cognitive processing practices. What this means is that each of us has learned over time to reach critical decisions by drawing upon varying amounts of relevant information and weighing up the relative costs and benefits of taking a specific action. This decision-making style is not determined by the individual's personality or intelligence, but might be conditioned by relevant learning experiences over their lifetime. These internal cognitive processes were also known to be associated with the perception of "fairness", which was poignant in the pandemic context because for some individuals, the restrictions on some of their behaviours, no matter how "just" the reasons for them might purport to be, were simply "unfair".

It is therefore relevant to understand how these internal cognitive processes can shape the way people think about crises that result in the imposition of severe restrictions on their behaviour. Some people would have weighed up many perspectives in reaching their own decision about compliance with pandemic-related restrictions, while others would have been influenced perhaps by only one argument or perspective, derived from a specific source. Each category of person would need a different approach in terms of persuasive campaigning designed to achieve behaviour change. While, "attitudes", "beliefs", "subjective norms", and "behavioural control" might all have represented important psychological precursors of behaviour change, not everyone will take all these factors into account when reaching a final decision about their own behaviour.

References

Ahmad, M., Iram, K., & Jabeen, G. (2020). Perception-based influence factors of intention to adopt COVID-19 epidemic prevention in China. *Environmental Research*, 190, 109995. https://doi.org/10.1016/j.envres.2020.109995

Ajzen, I. (1991). The theory of planned behavior. *Organisational Behavior and Human Decision Processes*, 50, 179–211. https://doi.org/10.1016/0749-5978(91)90020-T

Ajzen, I. (2001). Nature and operation of attitudes. *Annual Review of Psychology*, 52, 27–58. https://doi.org/10.1146/annurev.psych.52.1.27

Ajzen, I., & Kruglanski, A. W. (2019). Reasoned action in the service of goal pursuit. *Psychological Review*, 126, 74–86. https://doi.org/10.1037/rev0000155

Ajzen, I., & Madden, T. J. (1986). Prediction of goal-directed behavior: Attitudes, intentions, and perceived behavioral control. *Journal of Experimental Social Psychology*, 22, 453–474. https://doi.org/10.1016/0022-1031(86)90045-4

Al-Hasan, A., Yim, D., & Khuntia, J. (2020). Citizens' adherence to COVID-19 mitigation recommendations by the government: A 3-country comparative evaluation using web-based cross-sectional survey data. *Journal of Medicine and Internet Research*, 22(8), e20634. https://doi.org/10.2196/20634

Ammar, N., Aly, N. M., Folayan, M. O., Khader, Y., Virtanen, J. I., Al-Batayneh, O. B., et al. (2020). Behavior change due to COVID-19 among dental academics – the theory of planned behavior: Stresses, worries, training and pandemic severity. *PLoS One*. https://doi.org/10.1371/journal.pone.0239961

Andarge, E., Fikadu, T., Temesgen, R., Shegaze, M., Feleke, T., Haile, F., et al. (2020). Intention and practice on personal preventive measures against the covid-19 pandemic among adults with chronic conditions in southern Ethiopia: A survey using the theory of planned behavior. *Journal of Multidisciplinary Healthcare*, 13, 1863–1877. https://doi.org/10.2147/JMDH.S284707

Andrew, B. J., Mullan, B. A., de Wit, J. B. F., Monds, L. A., Todd, J., & Kothe, E. J. (2016). Does the theory of planned behaviour explain condom use behaviour among men who have sex with men? A meta-analytic review of the literature. *AIDS Behaviour*, 20, 834–844. https://doi.org/10.1007/s10461-016-1314-0

Armitage, C. J., & Conner, M. (2001). Efficacy of the theory of planned behaviour: A meta-analytic review. *British Journal of Social Psychology*, 40(4), 471–499. https://doi.org/10.1348/014466601164939

Arrow, K. J. (1971). Aspects of the theory of risk bearing. The theory of risk aversion. Helsinki: Yrjo Jahnssonin Saatio. In *Essays in the Theory of Risk Bearing* (pp. 90–109). Chicago: Markham Publishing Company.

Aschwanden, D., Strickhauser, J. E., Sesker, A. A., Lee, J.-Y., Luchetti, M., Terracciano, A., & Sutin, A. R. (2021). Preventive behaviors during the COVID-19 pandemic: Associations with perceived behavioral control, attitudes and subjective norms. *Frontiers in Public Health.* https://doi.org/10.3389/fpubh.2021.662835

Baddeley, A. D., & Hitch, G. (2020). Working memory. *Psychology of Learning and Motivation, 8,* 47–89.

Bandura, A. (1977). Self-efficacy: Toward a unifying theory of behavioral change. *Psychological Review, 84*(2), 191–215.

Bandura, A. (1978). Self-efficacy: Toward a unifying theory of behavioral change. *Advances in Behavior Research and Therapy, 1*(4), 139–161.

Barrett, C., & Cheung, K. L. (2021). Knowledge, socio-cognitive perceptions and the practice of hand hygiene and social distancing during the COVID-19 pandemic: A cross-sectional study of UK university students. *BMC Public Health, 21*(1), 426. doi: 10.1186/s12889-021-10461-0

Bogliacino, F., Codagnone, C., Montealegre, F., et al. (2021). Negative shocks predict change in cognitive function and preferences: Assessing the negative affect and stress hypothesis. *Science Reports, 11,* 3546. https://doi.org/10.1038/s41598-021-83089-0

Bowles, S., & Polanía-Reyes, S. (2012). Economic incentives and social preferences: Substitutes or complements? *Journal of Economic. Literature, 50*(2), 368–425.

Callow, M. A., Callow, D. D., & Smith, C. (2020). Older adults' intention to socially isolate once COVID-19 stay-at-home orders are replaced with "Safer-at-Home" public health advisories: A survey of respondents in Maryland. *Journal of Applied Gerontology, 39*(11), 1175–1183. doi: 10.1177/0733464820944704

Chan, D. K.-C., Yang, S. X., Mullan, B., Du, X., Zhang, X., Chatzisarantis, N. L. D., et al. (2015). Preventing the spread of H1N1 influenza infection during a pandemic: Autonomy-supportive advice versus controlling instruction. *Journal of Behavioural Medicine, 38,* 416–426.

Cheng, C., & Ng, A.-K. (2006). Psychosocial factors predicting SARS-preventive behaviors in four major SARS-affected regions. *Journal of Applied Social Psychology, 36,* 222–247.

Clark, C., Davila, A., Regis, M., & Kraus, S. (2020). Predictors of COVID-19 voluntary compliance behaviors: An international investigation. *Global Transitions, 2,* 76–82. doi: https://doi.org/10.1016/j.glt.2020.06.003

Cooke, R., Dahdah, M., Norman, P., & French, D. P. (2016). How well does the theory of planned behaviour predict alcohol consumption? A systematic review and meta-analysis. *Health Psychological Review, 10,* 148–167.

Coroiu, A., Moran, C., Campbell, T., & Geller, A. C. (2020). Barriers and facilitators to adherence to social distancing recommendations during COVID-19 among a large international sample of adults. *PLoS One, 15*(10), e0239795. https://doi.org/10.1371/journal.pone.0239795

Cowan, N. (2001). The magical number 4 in short-term memory: A reconsideration of mental storage capacity. *Behaviour and Brain Science, 24,* 87–114, discussion 114–185.

Curseu, P. L., Coman, A. D., Fodor, O. C., & Panchenko, A. (2021). Let's not joke about it too much! Exposure to COVID-19 messaging, attitudes and protective behavioral intentions. *Healthcare, 9*(2). https://doi.org/10.3390/healthcare902122

Das, A. K. et al. (2020). Fighting ahead: Adoption of social distancing in COVID-19 outbreak through the lens of theory of planned behaviour. *Journal of Human Behavior in the Social Environment, 31*(5). doi: 10.1080/10911359.2020.1833804

Diamond, A. (2013). Executive functions. *Annual Reviews of Psychology, 64*(1), 135–168.

Eagly, A. H., & Chaiken, S. (1993). *The Psychology of Attitudes*. New York, NY: Harcourt Brace Jovanovich College Publishers.

Frounfelker, R. L., Santavicca, T., Li, Z. Y., Miconi, D., Venkatesh, V., & Rousseau, C. (2021). COVID-19 experiences and social distancing: Insights from the theory of planned behaviour. *American Journal of Health Promotion, 2*, 8901171211020997. https://doi.org/10.1177/08901171211020997

Gibson, L. P., Magnan, R. E., Kramer, E. B., & Bryan, A. D. (2021). Theory of planned behaviour analysis of social distancing during the COVID-19 pandemic: Focusing on the intention-behaviour gap. *Annals of Behaviour and Medicine*. https://doi.org/10.1093/abm/kaab041

Grimes, M., & Marquardson, J. (2019). Quality matters: Evoking subjective norms and coping appraisals by system design to increase security intentions. *Decision Support Systems, 119*, 23–34.

Hagger, M. S., Smith, S. R., Keech, J. J., Moyers, S. A., & Hamilton, K. (2020). Predicting social distancing intention and behaviour during the COVID-19 pandemic: An integrated social cognition model. *Annals of Behaviour and Medicine, 54*(10), 713–727.

Ho, S. M., Ocasio-Velázquez, M., & Booth, C. (2017). Trust or consequences? Causal effects of perceived risk and subjective norms on cloud technology adoption. *Computers and Security, 70*, 581–595.

Huijsmans, I., Ma, I., Micheli, L., Civai, C., Stallen, M., & Sanfey, A. G. (2019). A scarcity mindset alters neural processing underlying consumer decision making. *Proceedings of the National Academy of Sciences of the United States of America, 116*, 11699–11704.

Kiriakidis, S. P. (2015). Theory of planned behaviour: The intention-behaviour relationship and the perceived behavioural control (PBC) relationship with intention and behaviour.

Lin, C., Imani, V., Majd, N. R., Ghasemi, Z., Griffiths, M. D., Hamilton, K., et al. (2020). Using an integrated social cognition model to predict COVID-19 preventive behaviours. *British Journal of Health Psychology, 25*, 981–1005.

Luck, S. J., & Vogel, E. K. (2013). Visual working memory capacity: From psychophysics and neurobiology to individual differences. *Trends in Cognitive Science, 17*(8), 391–400.

Mahardika, H., Thomas, D., Ewing, M. T., & Japutra, A. (2020). Comparing the temporal stability of behavioural expectation and behavioural intention in the prediction of consumers pro-environmental behaviour. *Journal of Retail and Consumer Services, 54*, 101943. https://doi.org/10.1016/j.jretconser.2019.101943

Mani, A., Mullainathan, S., Shafir, E., & Zhao, J. (2013). Poverty impedes cognitive function. *Science, 341*, 976–980.

Margraf, J., Brailovskaia, J., & Schneider, S. (2020). Behavioral measures to fight COVID-19: An 8-country study of perceived usefulness, adherence and their predictors. *PLoS One, 15*(12), e0243523. https://doi.org/10.1371/journal.pone.0243523

McDermott, M. S., Oliver, M., Simnadis, T., Beck, E. J., Coltman, T., Iverson, D., et al. (2015). The theory of planned behaviour and dietary patterns: A systematic review and meta-analysis. *Preventive Medicine, 81*, 150–156.

McEachan, R. R. C., Conner, M., Taylor, N. J., & Lawton, R. J. (2011). Prospective prediction of health-related behaviours with the theory of planned behaviour: A meta-analysis. *Health Psychology Review, 5*, 97–144.

McMillan, B., & Conner, M. (2003). Using the theory of planned behaviour to understand alcohol and tobacco use in students. *Psychology, Health and Medicine, 8*(3), 317–328.

Moore, R. C., Lee, A., Hancock, J. T., Halley, M., & Linos, E. (2020). Experience with social distancing early in the COVID-19 pandemic in the United States: Implications for public health messaging. *medRxiv* [Preprint]. Published 11 April 2020. https://doi.org/10.1101/2020.04.08.20057067

Mullainathan, S., & Shafir, E. (2014). *Scarcity: The True Cost of Not Having Enough*. New York, NY: Penguin.

Myyry, L., Siponen, M., Pahnila, S., Vartiainen, T., & Vance A. (2009). What levels of moral reasoning and values explain adherence to information security rules? An empirical study. *European Journal of Information Systems, 18*(2), 126–139.

Pahnila, S., Siponen, M., & Mahmood, A. (2007). Employees behaviour towards IS security policy compliance. *2007 40th Annual Hawaii International Conference on System Sciences (HICSS07)*. https://doi.org/10.1109/hicss.2007.206

Pan, Y., Fang, Y., Xin, M., Dong, W., Zhou, L., Hou, Q., et al. (2020). Self-reported compliance with personal preventive measures among Chinese factory workers at the beginning of work resumption following the covid-19 outbreak: cross-sectional survey study. *Journal of Medical Internet Research, 22*, e22457. https://doi.org/10.2196/22457

Prasetyo, Y. T., Castillo, A. M., Salonga, L. J., Sia, J. A., & Seneta, J. A. (2020). Factors affecting perceived effectiveness of COVID-19 prevention measures among Filipinos during enhanced community quarantine in Luzon, Philippines: Integrating protection motivation theory and extended theory of planned behavior. *International Journal of Infectious Diseases, 99*, 312–323.

Pratt, J. W. (1964). Risk aversion in the small and in the large. *Econometrica, 32*(1–2), 122–136.

Probst, T. M., Lee, H. J., & Bazzoli, A. (2020). Economic stressors and the enactment of CDC-recommended COVID-19 prevention behaviours: The impact of state-level context. *Journal of Applied Psychology, 105*(12), 1397–1407. https://doi.org/10.1037/apl0000797

Reluga, T. C. (2010). Game theory of social distancing in response to an epidemic. *PLoS Computational Biology, 6*, e1000793.

Rich, A., Brandes, K., Mullan, B., & Hagger, M. S. (2015). Theory of planned behavior and adherence in chronic illness: A meta-analysis. *Journal of Behavioural Medicine, 38*, 673–688. https://doi.org/10.1007/s10865-015-9644-3

Sasse, M., Brostoff, S., & Weirich, D. (2002). Transforming the weakest link: A human-computer interaction approach to usable and effective security. *Internet and Wireless Security*, 243–262. https://doi.org/10.1049/pbbt004e_ch15. Retrieved from: https://digital-library.theiet.org/content/books/10.1049/pbbt004e_ch15

Shah, A. K., Mullainathan, S., & Shafir, E. (2012). Some consequences of having too little. *Science*, *338*, 682–685. https://doi.org/10.1126/science.1222426

Sheeran, P., Trafimow, D., & Armitage, C. J. (2003). Predicting behaviour from perceived behavioural control: Tests of the accuracy assumption of the theory of planned behaviour. *British Journal of Social Psychology*, *42*(Pt 3), 393–410. doi: 10.1348/014466603322438224

Shubayr, M. A., Mashyakhy, M., Al Agili, D. E., Albar, N., & Quadri, M. F. (2020). Factors associated with infection-control behavior of dental health-care workers during the COVID-19 pandemic: A cross-sectional study applying the theory of planned behavior. *Journal of Multidisciplinary Healthcare*, *13*, 1527–1535. doi: https://doi.org/10.2147/JMDH.S278078

Starfelt Sutton, L. C., & White, K. M. (2016). Predicting sun-protective intentions and behaviours using the theory of planned behaviour: A systematic review and meta-analysis. *Psychology & Health*, *31*, 1272–1292. https://doi.org/10.1080/08870446.2016.1204449

Sturman, D., Auton, J. C., & Thacker, J. (2021). Knowledge of social distancing measures and adherence to restrictions during the COVID-19 pandemic. *Health Promotion Journal of Australia*, *32*(2), 344–351. https://doi.org/10.1002/hpja.443

Trifiletti, E., Shamloo, S. E., Faccini, M., & Zaka, A. (2021). Psychological predictors of protective behaviours during the Covid-19 pandemic: Theory of planned behaviour and risk perception. *Journal of Community & Applied Social Psychology*, Advance online publication. https://doi.org/10.1002/casp.2509

Williams, S. N., Armitage, C. J., Tampe, T., & Dienes, K. (2020). Public perceptions and experiences of social distancing and social isolation during the COVID-19 pandemic: A UK-based focus group study. *BMJ Open*, *10*(7), e039334. https://doi.org/10.1136/bmjopen-2020-039334

Workman, M., Bommer, W. H., & Straub, D. (2008). Security lapses and the omission of information security measures: A threat control model and empirical test. *Computers and Human Behaviour*, *24*(6), 2799–2816. https://doi.org/10.1016/j.chb.2008.04.005

Xia, Y., Shi, L. S., Chang, J. H., Miao, H. Z., & Wang, O. (2021). Impact of the COVID-19 pandemic on intention to use traditional Chinese medicine: A cross-sectional study based on the theory of planned behavior. *Journal of Integrative Medicine*. https://doi.org/10.1016/j.joim.2021.01.013

Xie, W., Campbell, S., & Zhang, W. (2020). Working memory capacity predicts individual differences in social-distancing compliance during the COVID-19 pandemic in the United States. *Proceedings of the National Academic of Sciences of the United States*, *117*(3), 17667–17774.

Yu, Y., Lau, J. T. F., & Lau, M. M. C. (2021). Levels and factors of social and physical distancing based on the theory of planned behavior during the COVID-19 pandemic among Chinese adults. *Translational Behavioural Medicine*, *11*(5), 1179–1186 [Epub ahead of print]. https://doi.org/10.1093/tbm/ibaa146

Zhang, K. C., Fang, Y., Cao, H., Chen, H., Hu, T., Chen, Y., et al. (2021). Behavioral intention to receive a covid-19 vaccination among Chinese factory workers: Cross-sectional online survey. *Journal of Medical Internet Research*, *23*, e24673. https://doi.org/10.2196/24673

Zhang, K. C., Fang, Y., Cao, H., Chen, H., Hu, T., Chen, Y. Q., et al. (2020). Parental acceptability of covid-19 vaccination for children under the age of 18 years: Cross-sectional online survey. *JMIR Pediatrics and Parenting*, *3*, e24827. https://doi.org/10.2196/24827

Zhang, W., & Luck, S. J. (2013). Discrete fixed-resolution representations in visual working memory. *Nature*, *453*, 233–235.

Chapter 9

COM-B Approach and Physical Distancing

On 3rd March 2020, the UK government released an action plan for how to cope with the novel coronavirus that had originated in China just a few months earlier but now had reached British shores and was known to spreading through the population at an accelerated pace. There was no known vaccine available to protect against infection and no tried-and-tested drug therapies for those infected. The remaining options for control of a burgeoning epidemic therefore were centred on public behaviour. There were a number of protective practices that could be recommended. Some of these focused on hygiene measures such as regular and thorough hand-washing after touching surfaces while moving around out of home, keeping surfaces clean in public spaces frequented by many people and coughing or sneezing into your elbow or a face covering. In addition, other public health protection techniques, effective with airborne diseases, involved keeping people physically apart from each other as much as possible, encouraging people to stay home and asking people to quarantine themselves if they become symptomatic with the virus. The UK government was initially reluctant to activate all these measures, but with weeks it had changed its strategy and imposed a wide range of behavioural restrictions on people.

Observations made during previous pandemics indicated that people would not always be willing to comply voluntarily with all these measures. While some would do so eventually, their uptake was often slow. Another factor was public awareness. The public did not always know what to do. If the information given out by government or public health authorities was sketchy or ambiguous, people might remain ignorant or confused and therefore no know what kinds of actions they could take that would protect them.

As previous chapters have discussed, when considered a psychological challenge, two theories in particular – nudge theory and the theory of panned behaviour – were widely used to provide guidance to public health strategy and planning under emergency conditions. Both of these theories were found to provide effective models of behaviour analysis and prediction of behavioural outcomes under some conditions. They were not perfect,

DOI: 10.4324/9781003274308-9

however, but then no theory is. Yet, it was also fair to say that even when they did predict certain behavioural outcomes or intentions on the part of people to adopt specific behaviours, neither theory provided a complete explanation of human behaviour choices.

Some psychologists critiqued these and other theoretical models that had been used in health behaviour change contexts and decided that a different approach was possible and that this approach might even provide more comprehensive accounts of people's behaviour change choices. This new model came to be known as the COM-B model. COM-B stands for capability-opportunity-motivation-behaviour (Michie et al., 2020). With capability, this embraces the idea that individuals must possess the knowledge and skill to perform specific behaviours. They may have a positive attitude towards the target behaviour, perceive that it is endorsed and performed by many other people, and believe that it is within the ability to perform.

Nudge theory relied on the use of subtle messages and signals placed in different environmental settings where behaviour change was sought. As a model, it represents a soft touch approach to behaviour because it leaves the final decision up to the individual. It encourages individuals to make their own judgements and draw their own conclusions about social situations that result in performance of a desired behaviour. Often, these judgements involve outcome or risk assessments by people themselves. Sometimes, the targeted behaviour is encouraged by markers and signs placed at appropriate points in an environment.

Group processes and social identity were envisaged to influence behaviour by creating ambient social conditions in which individuals would seek to behave in ways accepted, approved or normalised by others. These "others" would exert more influence over the individual's behavioural choice if the individual is identified with them or referenced them and their values and behaviour when defining their self-identity.

Within the theory of planned behaviour framework, attitudes and beliefs about the target behaviour and beliefs about the behaviour of others are important precursors to behaviour change. These variables were hypothesised to predict increased likelihood of the individual enacting the behaviour in question. Yet, regardless of their perceptions of others or themselves, ultimately, they must possess the capability to enact the behaviour. This means having the understanding of how and when to do so and the physical ability to do so. Then, the right opportunity must surface for the behaviour to take place. This is in part underpinned by whether others will allow them to perform a specific behaviour and also depends upon whether they have the resources for the behaviour.

Capability factors in relation to social distancing were defined principally by people knowing what they should do, when, where and how. Further support could then be provided in different environments through the use of signage and floor markings to remind people of the need to keep physically apart from others and to follow the lead of marks and signs designed to illustrate the kind of distance apart they should keep in specific settings (e.g., banks, cafes, supermarkets, etc.).

With opportunity, keeping the required physical distance apart should be clearly feasible within any space they enter. Following these rules, again, can be reinforced by signage. Seeing other people in compliance with the requirements will further reinforce the behaviour. The rate of footfall in specific physical spaces might have to be controlled to ensure they did not get too crowded and hence render maintenance of physical distancing more difficult. The movements of people around a space might also need to be controlled in some settings to guard against accidental breaches of physical distancing rules.

Finally, motivation to maintain physical distancing will be influenced by whether the behaviour is supported by individuals' attitudes and beliefs concerning the restrictions and identification with others who show either compliance or non-compliance. Signs and notices can be set up within physical spaces as reminders of the behaviour required and to help individuals remain compliant. Rejection of physical distancing restrictions, however, might weaken the impact of these environmental reminders.

From the outline above, it is clear that COM-B combines many of the defining elements of nudge theory (signage), planned behaviour (attitudes and beliefs) and group processes and social identity (self-identity and taking the lead from others) theories. Then it often adds other models into the mix.

The capability and opportunity factors can vary from one setting to another and this means that they need to be calibrated in ways that work for the scenario in which a target behaviour is expected to occur. Specific nudges might be expected to work in different settings. Internal rationalising constructs will tend to be measured by the theory of planned behaviour in fairly standard ways across settings. COM-B recognises that a more pragmatic approach that attempts to tailor research, from the types of theoretical constructs considered through to the way these constructs are operational defined or measured in practice, to suit the occasion. A key starting point therefore is to be very clear about the behaviour changes that you want to make. Understand the circumstances under which this will or is likely to happen. Then, more detailed aspects of research design flow from that point.

The COM-B model also regards the participants in research as representatives of a wider population. The behaviour changes being investigated might be expected to occur across an entire population. It is important to understand what works with individuals. Hence, research is more than a theoretical exercise attempting to validate a specific theoretical model. It is about finding solutions to problems that work in the real world. This is vitally important when research is being used to gather intelligence to guide public policy and strategies designed to protect people from a real crisis situation in which lives could be lost if the wrong decisions are made.

In this context, the proponents of the COM-B model recommended that individuals can enhance their capability through learning how to enact specific behaviours and by practising them to perform them better. Hence, as a construct, capability is not fixed in stone. It is fluid. Turning to opportunity, individuals and policy makers can bring this construct under their control through forward planning and by establishing that all requisite steps have been taken to facilitate a specific behaviour when the time comes for it to be displayed. Boosting motivation to perform a behaviour does not just depend on capability and opportunity but can be further enhanced if the behaviour itself is made attractive and socially acceptable as an appropriate course of action to take.

Examples have been provided of how this approach would work in the context of the COVID-19 pandemic. For example, keeping hands thoroughly washed means understanding that soap and sanitiser can be used but that specific behavioural practices must be followed such as washing for long enough, washing the backs of hands as thoroughly as the palms and washing between the fingers. When it comes to avoidance of social gatherings, it might be important to plan routes when moving from one location to another or changes the usual times for visiting specific locations (e.g., supermarkets) to when they are less busy. The critical observation here as far the COVID-19 pandemic is concerned is that when lockdown restrictions were deployed, this was totally a new experience practically for the entire population of most countries. This meant that the kind of advanced planning being described here did not exist in the behaviour repertoires of most people.

Hence, in testing the efficacy of behaviour change strategies, it is important to build into research protocols some ideas about how any new understanding discovered by research can be translated into actionable behaviour for members of the public. There will also be psychological costs of extreme restrictions on public behaviour, especially when the restrictions create conditions of social deprivation. Some individuals will cope better than others with these conditions. Some will not cope well at all. Helping everybody and most of all those with poorer coping mechanisms is essential to restrict lasting social and psychological damage to societies when they use extreme measures to bring out of control pandemics under control.

One set of recommendations outlined by Michie et al. (2020) included the following principles:

- Practice developing the skills required.
- Establish routines and *habits*.
- Make the changes as *easy* as possible.

- Make *plans* including how to overcome possible barriers to the behaviours.
- Ask for *support* and *feedback* from family, friends and colleagues.
- If you are doing less of things you enjoy, try to find *enjoyable alternatives*.

COM-B and Beyond Nudging, Social Identity and Planned Behaviour

The capabilities, opportunities, motivation, behaviour (COM-B) model was derived from a systematic review of a wide range of psychological theories and empirical analyses of human behaviour (Michie et al., 2011). It was adopted within the United Kingdom as a core framework for defining strategies for controlling public behaviour during the COVID-19 pandemic (Gibson Miller et al., 2020).

Capability was in turn defined in terms of having the knowledge and physical ability to change behaviour. Opportunity was articulated in terms of the presence of relevant social and physical conditions to promote and support behaviour change. Motivation comprised an inner drive to change that was further underpinned by cognitive reasoning and emotional states, impulses and desires (Michie et al., 2014). These constructs can have individual effects on behaviour and can work together to have interactive or cumulative influences (Howlett et al., 2019; Wilkie et al., 2018).

Specific components of the COM-B model predicted the likelihood that physical activity levels would improve in the future. Principally, the perception of the physical opportunity to exercise and the motivation to make the effort to do so were critical (Spence et al., 2020). According to this model, understanding how to change behaviours depends on the following core constructs: capability, opportunity and motivation. In a UK study of people's activity levels during the pandemic, over half of a national sample (57%) said they had maintained or increased their physical activity during the pandemic, but fewer than a third (31%) were exercising enough to meet national guidelines (Spence et al., 2020).

An online survey obtained responses from 649 respondents and revealed that people's knowledge and understanding of COVID-19 had no direct effects on their perceived vulnerability or on how serious they believed this disease could be. Following the theory of planned behaviour model, measures were taken of attitude, subjective norm and perceived behavioural control, as well as of perceived vulnerability to and perceived severity of the new disease. Measures were also taken of intention to comply with recommended or required behaviours and whether these behaviours were actually adopted.

Perceived severity of and personal vulnerability to COVID-19 had some indirect influence on people's intention to follow behavioural restrictions. In particular, understanding of how COVID-19 could be caught, what to do if they caught it, and where there were hospitals offering treatment for this disease were all aspects of understanding about COVID-19. Better educated and better-off people in urban areas tended to exhibit better knowledge of COVID-19. Those who intended to follow the rules were also the ones who were in the end most likely to comply in actuality. The latter included restricting their behaviour where needed and adopting new protective behaviours where they were recommended.

It was concluded by the researchers that there could have been subjective norm and behavioural control effects at play as well. Better understanding should in theory have empowered people to know what to do and what it was feasible to do in relation to this disease. Further, if they were living in a community surrounded by many others who were behavioural compliant, they might be expected to confirm to similar behaviour patterns. In fact, their findings showed that perceived behavioural control was a significant predictor of intention to follow the rules. Subjective norm perceptions and positive attitudes towards restrictive behaviours also predicted intention to conform to behavioural restrictions, as expected under the theory of planned behaviour. Strengthening intention to behave was a positive result because this could in turn motivate actual compliance.

Research was also conducted on health professionals and their willingness to comply with new COVID-related procedures at work, underpinned by the planned behaviour model. One such study was conducted with 324 dental health-care workers in Saudi Arabia. Respondents' intentions to comply with relevant COVID-19 restrictions designed to control spread of infections were underpinned to some degree by having positive attitudes about whether this would be a good thing to do. The perception that others, especially relevant others, would also be compliant represented a further motivation of intention of respondents to be compliant themselves. Other moderating variables from this model such as general beliefs about the efficacy of the interventions or respondents' perceptions of their ability to comply were not significant predictors of intention to comply (Shubayr et al., 2020).

Framing Compliance within the COM-B Model

The COM-B model has been tested in the context of COVID-19. One study investigated its usefulness as a model for understanding whether people adopted specific hygiene practices designed to control infection transmission. Data were collected through a longitudinal survey, which began during the early phase of the pandemic in the United Kingdom (Miller et al., 2020). The study asked participants to indicate their motivation to adopt these behaviours and their capability and opportunity to do so.

The results revealed that all three of the C-O-M components emerged as significant statistical predictors of hygiene practices. Using a regression model to establish the relative predictive strengths of each of the model's core components, motivation emerged as having the strongest influence on behaviour. Further analysis found that capability and opportunity were also significant predictors of target behaviour outcomes. In conclusion, the researchers stated that interventions that are deigned to change people's health or hygiene behaviour need to focus on creating relevant motivation and effective performance of these measures. Adoption tends also to be underpinned by an understanding of way such measures are needed together with confidence in their proven effectiveness (Bavel et al., 2020; West et al., 2020).

The COM-B model outlines a range of psychological variables that are critical in an analysis of behaviour change. The model recognises internal (psychological) and external (environmental settings and stimulus) factors at play and understanding their specific effects and the overall impact of the interplay between them lies at the roots of this analytical model. In changing their behaviour, individuals must be able to do so both physically and psychologically largely by knowing what they have to do and why.

Then, individuals must have the opportunity to undertake the change. Finally, they must have the internal drives, cognitive and emotional, needed to make the behaviour happen and determine the form it will take (Michie et al., 2020). In explaining this model, Michie, West and Harvey developed a Behaviour Change Wheel (BCW), which displays the variables that needed to be measured and manipulated to drive a specific behaviour change forward (Michie et al., 2014). Initial diagnosis of the behaviour change objectives is undertaken to define the key variables to be incorporated in the analysis of a specific behaviour.

In the COVID-19 context, a range of behaviour changes were asked or demanded of the public. There were personal protective behaviours such as hand hygiene and face mask wearing. There were social distancing rules such as keeping a distance of two metres between self and others when visiting physical environments to carry out essential tasks such as food shopping. These behaviours were regarded by public health authorities as being essential to reducing transmission of this new virus (Walker et al., 2020; Moore et al., 2021). Ultimately, people would be protected from this new virus by vaccines but these were not available at the outset of the pandemic.

One of the big challenges with social distancing restrictions was just how long people would be willing and able to put up with them. The public showed extensive support for these measures at the outset (Duffy & Allington, 2020; Fancourt et al., 2020; Hale et al., 2020). Over time, however, motivation to keep going with these restrictions weakened for some (Bavel et al., 2020). This was always a concern and initially discouraged the United Kingdom's authorities from implementing full "lockdown". Repeated lockdowns could also seriously test the resolve of the public to stick with these behavioural restrictions. Other priorities could surface that would tempt people to engage in rule breaches, especially where these concerned interactions were with family members (Baumeister & Leary, 1995). Continued confidence in government was also essential (Wright et al., 2020). If the public began to question the competence or integrity of government and public health authorities, adherence to social distancing rules would certainly weaken.

Large-scale surveys showed that although most people did try to be compliant, there were still sizeable minorities that did not – or at least not always (Duffy & Allington, 2020). There could be a real challenge for some people if their homes provided a very limited setting in which to isolate. In some households, social isolation meant that family members were forced to spend more time together and this could result in internal tensions. The home might not have provided a comfortable working environment. In large households with many members extended across generations, some of which were classed as "high risk" for infection, the opportunities for wider spread of the disease were increased. So, for disadvantaged groups, lockdown was a far from pleasant experience (Marmot, 2020).

The COVID-19 Psychological Research Consortium (C19PRC) Study group of researchers conducted longitudinal and international research across the four UK nations and compared the data with research in Ireland, Italy, Spain and Saudi Arabia. They used the COM-B model to analyse and interpret the findings. They measured participants' motivations, capability and opportunity to perform specific self-protective behaviours. It was the second of two surveys that asked respondents questions about compliance with social distancing rules (Gibson-Miller et al., 2021).

Participants were asked about their propensity to engage with a number of described behaviours such as close physical contact when greeting people (e.g., hand-shaking), keeping two metres apart from people when meeting the indoors; meeting in a group of more than two people in a park. All the behaviours described were technically in breach of current COVID rules. Only psychological capability was a significant predictor or social distancing compliance, although older people and those who lived in urban locations also displayed more psychological capability. Once again, women showed a stronger tendency to be motivated to comply with social distancing than did men.

A further survey wave continued to collect data about longer-term adherence to social distancing rules in December 2020. The researchers asked participants "...how willing you are to break rules or conventions". Five items were presented: "I have driven a car at more than 10 miles an hour"; "I have travelled illegally to North Korea"; "I have sometimes not paid my bills on time"; "I have borrowed something from a friend and forgotten to return it"; and "I have socialised in another household during lockdown". The last item was the critical one. The research showed that one in four people said they had violated government guidelines by socialising with people from another household when they should not have done. Data were also collected about participant's anxiety levels and those who were more anxious were also most likely to follow the rules (Gibson-Miller et al., 2021).

With physical distancing, it was important to focus on the public's beliefs about their psychological capability to comply and this could be reinforced by better knowledge about why social distancing was important. Some population sub-groups reportedly experienced barriers to compliance because, for various reasons, they felt unable to comply. For some, the challenges to compliance were purely psychological and for others it might be linked to economic reasons (e.g., job loss, fall in income) or physical reasons (e.g., insufficient space in household to work or tensions in crowded households with everyone home at the same time). Public policies would be needed, tailored to these groups, to render social distancing more doable (Gibson-Miller et al., 2021).

Research with people living in Europe and North America between the end of March and mid-April 2020 investigated motivations to engage in social distancing practices. For most people, a prime motive for compliance with this behaviour was a sense of social responsibility "to protect others" (86%), and this was further re-enforced by almost as many (84%) saying that they felt a sense of responsibility towards their community. Most (84%) also wanted to protect themselves. For one in four respondents (25%) one challenge that confronted them was that they had to run errands for family members and friends during the pandemic and this behaviour presumably meant that they had to venture out more than they would have done otherwise. Manifestations of social distancing most often reported by these samples mostly comprised working from home and avoidance of crowded places. Men and young people (aged 18–24 years) tended to report less compliance with social distancing than did women and older people (Coroiu et al., 2020).

In a UK study of public compliance with a range of COVID-19 related interventions, which was one of series of analyses on data from the UCL COVID-19 Social Study, evidence emerged that social distancing (along with other measures such as amount of indoor and outdoor household mixing) attracted high levels of compliance (with more than 80% saying they frequently or occasionally complied). Social distancing achieved the highest level of compliance among just under half, meaning that there remained many people that complied, but not always. Compliance was lower among younger people, those who were risk takers, who had poor empathy, and had less confidence in the government (Wright et al., 2021a).

In a further study by the same research group, higher self-reported compliance with social distancing (and other interventions) was associated with having greater confidence in government. There was little significant evidence that social isolation, loneliness and mental health or well-being were linked to propensity to comply (Wright et al., 2021b).

The COM-B model underpinned the interpretation of findings from semi-structured interviews with a small sample of UK adults ($n = 116$) about their compliance with social distancing rules. The aim of this study was to identify barriers to and facilitators of compliance. The findings showed that the capability, opportunity and motivation components of this model were all relevant in explaining whether people taking part had complied or not with social distancing (Burton et al., 2020).

Key barriers mentioned by these interviewees were inconsistent rules, having caring responsibilities, fatigue, unintended consequences of the COVID interventions and a need for more emotional support. There was evidence also that the behaviour of others could make a difference. In terms of motivation, perceptions of self-risk of infection, concern about infection of others, direct experiences of COVID-19, caring responsibilities for others, especially children, and a wide sense of social concern were identified by interviewees as occupying their thoughts about how to behave.

Having good information was also linked to how much trust was placed in government as the principal information source. At the time of this research, interviewees were still mindful of the behaviour of the prime minister's senior advisor, Dominic Cummings, who had breached the travel rules imposed during the pandemic. This undermined the confidence of some of them in the government.

Under opportunity, some people faced challenges with compliance with social distancing rules because they lived in homes with many others and their homes were situated in settings where complete avoidance of others even in surrounding public areas could be difficult. The need to visit pharmacies and supermarkets for essential items also meant some exposure to risk from others because it was rare to enter these spaces with no one else around. Psychologically, the opportunity to be compliant became psychologically constrained if others with whom an individual identified were not compliant.

The capability of individuals to comply depended upon whether they were sufficiently informed so as to know what they should do. This meant knowing what to do when shielding, when isolating and when go out and about for exercise or to buy essential items. It was also important that other people were seen to behave in consistent ways.

Behavioural fatigue was also recognised by these researchers as an explanation of non-compliance, despite this notion having been challenged by others (Harvey, 2020; Michie et al., 2020). It was identified by advisers to government in the United Kingdom during the period prior to the first lockdown as a problem for extreme measures positing that many people would quickly lose the will to remain compliant (Mahase, 2020). Yet, later studies found that publics' willingness to stay within extreme behavioural restrictions could wane over time (Wright et al., 2021c). One factor, already mentioned, that could further feed into this process was witnessing those in authority not following the rules themselves (Wright et al., 2021a).

Lessons Learned

Michie and West (2021) observed that human behaviour had been the key to controlling the COVID-19 pandemic. Governments around the world put their economics and societies on hold and managed to persuade their populations to engage with sweeping behaviour changes. In some instances, behaviour change was forced upon people with the compulsory closure of physical spaces in which they would normally interact. In others, voluntary compliance, with some legal enforcement, was engaged and people took it upon themselves to comply with government advice even though it could be painful both economically and psychologically.

Governments deployed a wide range of interventions, some medical, some behavioural and other economic to exert a degree of centralised control over their citizens' behaviour. These interventions were not used consistently around the world and varied in their relative effectiveness in terms of bringing virus transmission rates under control. These measures included advising or requiring people to stay home, to maintain a minimum physical distance between themselves and others when out and about, controls over large public gatherings, closures of leisure facilities, schools and non-essential shops, border controls, testing people for infection, quarantining those with the disease or those known to have been in close contact with the infected, wearing face masks, washing hands regularly, development of vaccines, among many others.

The COM-B model forecast that if people possess the capability and opportunity to change their behaviour, then they will be motivated to do so and behaviour change then becomes increasingly likely to occur. The behaviour change itself has a feedback loop to capability each of the other three components confirming the occurrence and therefore the feasibility of that change. The presence of specific interventions during the pandemic provided a backdrop to the determination of whether behaviour change was feasible in terms of capability and opportunity.

When pandemic-related restrictions required or advised people to stay at home, this behaviour change would have been more feasible for some than for others. For those people on low wages and with little or no savings, any change that reduced or completely removed their ability to earn would have placed them in severe difficulty. This state of affairs could be especially serious for those individuals with dependents. Ongoing costs of maintaining a home, putting food on the table, and making payments on loans would be put at risk if the individual's income stream suddenly dried up for many weeks or months. Many governments responded to this situation by providing partial cover for lost income out of public funds. Even so, many people suffered significant loss of income and a few did not qualify for these government payments at all. For those this might have meant losing their home, there would have been a temptation to ignore the advice or requirements which would probably have grown stronger the longer the restrictions prevailed.

For those working in critical care sectors such as the health and social care services, they had to continue working as normal. This meant that they were also confronted with enhanced personal risk of infection. It was essential in this context that these workers received adequate training and support to stay safe (capability concerns), that they were provided with safe spaces in which to work by their employers (opportunity concerns) and then finally that individuals trusted their employers, the government and the safety measures put in place (motivational factors) (Houghton et al., 2020).

The people needed to see that the government and others in authority had competence to deal with the crisis and made sensible decisions concerning ongoing problems. This would generate greater public trust and therefore a willingness to act upon the advice their government gave them. It was important that they identified with those advising them and accepted that everyone was "in this together". Any indications that those in government or authority did not always take their own advice or observe the rules they had imposed upon others could have a disastrous effect on public trust (Wright et al., 2020).

For Michie and West (2021), it was imperative that all these issues continued to be researched to enhance understanding. Events could move quickly during the pandemic. The massive quantity of research that had been funded by government meant that knowledge was growing apace and sometimes the "truths" that had been believed in the early phases of the pandemic changed with new findings coming down the research pipeline.

References

Baumeister, R. F., & Leary, M. R. (1995). The need to belong: Desire for interpersonal attachments as a fundamental human motivation. *Psychological Bulletin*, *117*(3), 497–529. https://doi.org/10.1037/0033-2909.117.3.497

Bavel, J. J. V., Baicker, K., Boggio, P. S., Capraro, V., Cichocka, A., Cikara, M., Crockett, M. J., Crum, A. J., Douglas, K. M., Druckman, J. N., Drury, J., Dube, O., Ellemers, N., Finkel, E. J., Fowler, J. H., Gelfand, M., Han, S., Haslam, S.A., Jetten, J., Kitayama, S., ... (2020). Using social and behavioural science to support COVID-19 pandemic response. *Nature and Human Behaviour*, *4*(5), 460–471. https://doi.org/10.1038/s41562-020-0884-z

Burton, A., McKinlay, A., Dawes, I., Roberts, A., Fynn, W., May, T., & Fancourt, D. (2020). Understanding barriers and facilitators to compliance with UK social distancing guidelines during the COVID-19 pandemic: A qualitative interview study. *PsyArXiv* Preprint. Retrieved from: https://psyarxiv.com/k4wqh/

Coroiu, A., Moran, C., Campbell, T., & Geller, A. C. (2020). Barriers and facilitators of adherence to social distancing recommendations during COVID-19 among a large international sample. *PloS One*. Retrieved from: https://journals.plos.org/plosone/article?id=10.1371/journal.pone.0239795

Duffy, B., & Allington, D. (2020). The accepting, the suffering and the resisting: The different reactions to life under lockdown. The Policy Institute, Kings College London. https://www.kcl.ac.uk/policy-institute/assets/Coronavirus-in-the-UK-cluster-analysis.pdf

Fancourt, D., Bu, F., Mak, H., & Steptoe, P. (2020). UCL Social Study Results Release 22. Available at: https://b6bdcb03-332c-4ff9-8b9d-28f9c957493a.filesusr.com/ugd/3d9db5_636933e8191d4783866c474fab3ca23

Gibson-Miller, J., Zavlis, O., Hartman, T. K., McBride, O., Bennett, K., Butter, S., Levita, L., Mason, L., Martinez, A. P., McKay, R., Murphy, J., Shevlin, M., Stocks, T. V. A., & Bentall, R. P. (2021). Psychological factors influencing protective behaviours during the COVID-19 pandemic: Capability, opportunity and motivation. In F. Gabrielli & F. Irtelli (Eds.), *Anxiety, Uncertainty, and Resilience during the Pandemic Period – Anthropological and Psychological Perspectives* (online ahead of print). Intech Open. https://doi.org/10.5772/intechopen.98237

Hale, T., Webster, S., Petherick, A., Phillips, T., & Kira, B. (2020). *Oxford COVID-19 Government Response Tracker*. Oxford, UK: Blavatnik School of Government, University of Oxford.

Harvey, N. (2020). Behavioural fatigue: Real phenomenon, naïve construct or policy contrivance? *Frontiers in Psychology, 11*(2960). https://doi.org/10.3389/fpsyg.2020.589892

Houghton, C. et al. (2020). *Cochrane Database of Systematic Reviews*, https://doi.org/10.1002/14651858.CD013582

Howlett, N., Schulz, J., Trivedi, D., Troop, N., & Chater, A. (2019). A prospective study exploring the construct and predictive validity of the COM-B model for physical activity. *Journal of Health Psychology, 24*, 1378–1391. https://doi.org/10.1177/1359105317739098

Mahase, F. (2020). Covid-19: Was the decision to delay the UK's lockdown over fears of "behavioural fatigue" based on evidence? *BMJ, 37*, M3166. https://doi.org/10.1136/bmj/M3166

Marmot, M. (2020). Society and the slow burn of inequality. *Lancet. 395*(10234), 1413–1414. https://doi.org/10.1016/S0140-6736(20)30940-5

Michie, S., Atkins, L., & West, R. (2014). *The Behaviour Change Wheel: A Guide to Designing Interventions*. London, UK: Silverback Publishing.

Michie, S., van Stralen, M. M., & West, R. (2011). The behaviour change wheel: A new method for characterising and designing behaviour change interventions. *Implementation Science, 6*(1), 42. https://doi.org/10.1186/1748-5908-6-4

Michie, S., & West, R. (2021). Sustained behavior change is key to preventing and tackling future pandemics. *Nature Medicine, 27*,749–752.

Michie, S., West, R., & Harvey, N. (2020). The concept of "fatigue" in tackling covid-19. *BMJ. 371*. https://doi.org/10.1136/bmj.m4171

Michie, S., West, R., & Smlot, R. (2020, 3rd March). Behavioural strategies for reducing covid-19 transmission in the general population. *thebmjopinion*. Retrieved from: https://blogs.bmj.com/bmj/2020/03/03/behavioural-strategies-for-reducing-covid-19-transmission-in-the-general-population/

Miller, J. G., Hartman, T. K., Levita, L., Martinez, A. P., Mason, L., McKay, R., Murphy, J., Shevlin, M., Stocks, T. V. A., Bennett, K. M., & Bentall, R. P. (2020). Capability, opportunity, and motivation to enact hygiene practices in the early stages of the COVID-19 outbreak in the United Kingdom. *British Journal of Health Psychology, 25*(4), 856–864.

Moore, S., Hill, E. M., Tildesley, M. J., Dyson, L., & Keeling, M. J. (2021). Vaccination and non-pharmaceutical interventions: When can the UK relax about COVID-19? *Medrxiv.* https://www.medrxiv.org/content/10.1101/2020.12.27.202488

Shubayr, M. A., Mashyakhy, M., Al Agili, D. E., Albar, N., & Quadri, M. F. (2020). Factors associated with infection-control behavior of dental health-care workers during the COVID-19 pandemic: A cross-sectional study applying the theory of planned behavior. *Journal of Multidisciplinary Healthcare, 13,*1527–1535. doi: https://doi.org/10.2147/JMDH.S278078

Spence, J., Rhodes, R. E., McCurdy, A., Mangan, A., Hopkins, D., & Mummery, W. K. (2020). Determinants of physical activity among adults in the United Kingdom during the COVID-19 pandemic: The DUK-COVID study. *British Journal of Health Psychology, 26*(2), 588–605.

Walker, P. G. T., Whittaker, C., Watson, O. J., Baguelin, M., Winstall, P., et al. (2020). The impact of COVID-19 and strategies for mitigation and suppression in middle- and low-income countries. *Science, 369*(6502), 413–422. https://doi.org/10.1126/science.abc0035

West, R., Michie, S., Rubin, G. J., & Amlôt, R. (2020). Applying principles of behaviour change to reduce SARS-CoV-2 transmission. *Nature and Human Behaviour, 4*(5), 451–459. https://doi.org/10.1038/s41562-020-0887-9

Wilkie, S., Townshend, T., Thompson, E., & Ling, J. (2018). Restructuring the built environment to change adult health behaviours: A scoping review integrated with behaviour change frameworks. *Cities & Health, 2*(2), 198– 211. https://doi.org/1 0.1080/23748834.2019.1574954

Wright, K., Steptoe, A., & Fancourt, D. (2020). What predicts adherence to COVID-19 government guidelines? Longitudinal analyses of 51,000 UK adults. *medRxiv.* https://doi.org/10.1101/2020.10.19.20215376

Wright, L., Steptoe, A., & Fancourt, D. (2021a). Patterns of compliance with COVID-19 preventive behaviours: A latent class analysis of 20,000 UK adults. *medRxiv.* https://doi.org/2021.2003.201621255717

Wright, L., Steptoe, A., & Fancourt, D. (2021b). Predictors of self-reported adherence to COVID-19 guidelines: A longitudinal observational study of 51,600 UK adults. *The Lancet.* https://doi.org/10.1016/j.lanepe.2021.100061

Wright, L., Steptoe, A., & Fancourt, D. (2021c). Trajectories of compliance with COVID-19 related guidelines: Longitudinal analysis of 50,000 UK adults. *medRxiv.* https://doi.org/10.1101/2021.04.13.21255336. https://www.medrxiv.org/content/10.1101/2021.04.13.21255336v1

Chapter 10

Ongoing Behavioural Interventions: Adoption of Personal Protection Measures

Many of the non-pharmaceutical interventions (NPIs) deployed by governments under advice from their public health authorities and other scientists comprised restrictions on physical behaviours and activities that were designed to keep most people apart in a real physical sense. This meant that tight restrictions were imposed by law on socialising between people from different households and, in many instances, it also meant compulsory closure of many public spaces such as schools and other educational establishments, hospitality and leisure venues, most retail outlets and most workplaces. In addition, there were two other sets of interventions – one pharmaceutical and another non-pharmaceutical. The former comprised the development of vaccines to protect people against catching or become seriously ill from COVID-19. The second comprised other protective measures linked to personal hygiene (regular handwashing and washing down of surfaces that might be touched by different people) and wearing face coverings to reduce airborne spread of the disease.

There was a lot of debate about face masks and their efficacy in protecting wearers from becoming infected. Masks are made of different materials and some of these are more porous than others when it comes to providing an effective barrier that is impervious to the coronavirus. Modelling work from the Far East has indicated that increased mask use in association with social distancing measures could help to flatten rising COVID-19 infection curves (Li et al., 2020). The researchers do make reference to the wearing of quality masks, therefore recognising that not all face masks are equally effective. Moreover, their results derive from modelling work in which face mask wearing was combined with social distancing which itself is potentially represented by a whole range of different interventions.

Another international study showed how the wearing of face masks was significantly associated with less face touching, known to be a primary route for the entry of many infections into humans. Research carried out in Asia (China, Japan, and South Korea), Europe (England, France, Germany, Italy and Spain) and the United States during 2018 and 2019 and again in

DOI: 10.4324/9781003274308-10

March 2020 during the COVID-19 pandemic investigated face touching behaviour and how this was related to mask wearing (Chen et al., 2020). Video evidence was used to observe people in different settings. Among those observed, rates of mask wearing were found to have increased from pre-pandemic periods to the pandemic period in Asia and Europe but not the United States. At the same time, face touching behaviours decreased. China departed somewhat from other countries in showing a significantly higher use of surgical masks that provided better protection than standard fabric masks. Comparing country by country, the more people wore face masks the progressively less often they were likely to touch their faces.

During the course of the COVID-19 pandemic, many national health authorities revisited the scientific evidence concerning the effectiveness of face masks. Masks and face covering visors had become integral pieces of protective kit for frontline health workers confronted with treating patients infected with the new coronavirus (Howard et al., 2021). It became apparent, however, that face masks might also be used by the wider population to protect others (from their own virus shedding) and therefore (if everyone joined in) also protecting themselves. The reasons for adoption of this protective measure needed to be explained to people to win over their compliance. For people in Western societies, face mask wearing was a new behaviour and no one was comfortable about (Song et al., 2020).

The use of face masks also opened up the opportunity for other NPIs, such as social distancing, to be modified in the way they were used. This could be important for certain businesses that could not operate on an economically viable basis under strict social distancing rules. If these businesses, and especially those in catering, could admit more people onto their premises than permitted under baseline social distancing restrictions, if their customer wore face masks, which provided an additional line of protection, they could become both economically more viable and do so without posing a significantly increased infection spread risk.

One of the main benefits of face mask wearing is that it can reduce the spread of an airborne virus even by people that are asymptomatic and therefore unaware that they are carrying the disease, and yet they remain infectious to others (Chu et al., 2020). The World Health Organization recognised that face masks could be useful in settings where other mitigating factors against the spread of airborne respiratory diseases were difficult to implement (World Health Organization, 2020).

Adoption of Protective Measures

Public adoption of NPIs could be influenced by many psychological variables. Among the important precursors were pandemic-related risk perceptions and knowledge. In China, adoption of interventions such as handwashing, hygienic coughing habits, face mask wearing and social distancing were more likely to occur among people with positive attitudes towards these behaviours, recognition of their importance and their ability to reduce disease risks. Further evidence confirmed that those who observed handwashing, good coughing hygiene, wore face masks and engaged in social distancing were in the end less likely to become infected with COVID-19. Face mask wearing could be especially effective in this regard (Xu et al., 2020).

Research with American women during May and June 2020 found a number of factors that predicted compliance with recommended protective measures. Women from urban environments with poorer education and a lower household income were less likely to comply with pandemic-related interventions and this included the propensity to wear face masks (Anderson & Stockmarr, 2021).

The propensity to comply with specific behavioural interventions was found to be widespread in most countries. Yet, some NPIs were better received and more extensively adopted than others. Further, some sub-groups in the population, defined for instance by their demography and culture, were also more likely to comply and others not to do so (Allcott et al., 2020; Berg & Lin, 2020; Harper et al., 2020; Plohl & Musil, 2020).

Population Sub-group Variances

The population sub-group differences in compliance with COVID-19 prevention behaviours varied between different types of behavioural restriction. Some groups had difficulty being compliant with stay-at-home orders because they could not afford to take time off work or risk of losing their jobs. Another barrier to compliance was whether workers did essential jobs in the health and social care services and for understandable reasons were expected to continue to go to their regular place of employment because the nature of their work meant they could not do it remotely. These problems were found to be especially serious for some ethnic minority groups (Centers for Disease Control and Prevention Coronavirus Disease 2019: Racial & Ethnic Minority Groups, 2020; Kantamneni, 2020; Poteat et al., 2020).

The level of education attained by people in different communities emerged as a predictor of use of face coverings. Better educated people were more likely to be compliant. This was not a new finding. It had also been previously found to make a difference to behaviour change in earlier health settings (Berkman et al., 2011). Some researchers concluded that people chose the prevention behaviours they felt most readily able to accommodate in their own lives (Cowling et al., 2020; West et al., 2020).

Elsewhere, research found that women who knew where to get tested for COVID-19 had a much greater likelihood than those ignorant of this to wear face masks. One possible explanation of this difference might be that those with greater broader awareness about pandemic-related protective behaviours were better informed about the benefits of wearing face masks (Razzaghi et al., 2020).

Another factor of significance here is that women have typically exhibited greater fear about chronic health conditions and therefore could be expected to take more pandemic-related precautions than men for that reason. Researchers have also debated whether the use of fear as a motivator of behaviour change in this context is a good idea. There is mixed evidence on whether it is effective and there is also evidence that it can trigger unwelcome side effects, especially in relation to people's mental health (Bradley et al., 2020; Fitzpatrick et al., 2020; Tannenbaum et al., 2015).

Greater household income emerged as a generic factor that was related to better general health literacy. This, in turn, was related to a greater likelihood of behavioural compliance. Lower income individuals might also be confronted with a problem with face masks because they could not afford to keep buying them (Berkman et al., 2011).

Compliance with COVID-19 safety measures can vary from one person to the next. It can also vary between communities. Pandemic-related interventions could only be effective in slowing the spread of the new virus if people complied with them. Evidence emerged from behavioural science studies that non-compliance was more likely to occur where opportunities to break the rules were more prevalent (Ngonghala et al., 2020). In the United States, for instance, the governments of individual states varied in the degree to which they mandated compliance with specific interventions such as face mask wearing and social distancing (Haffajee & Mello, 2020). Hence, in some states, where interventions were recommended but not required by law, voluntary public compliance was crucial.

A study in the United States found that women (and men) who had displayed stronger propensities to think about their physical appearance, who were anxious about being judged on this basis and who also exhibited stronger anxieties about their physical safety were also more inclined to comply with many COVID-19 restrictions and interventions, especially those which required them to think about their physical state (e.g., personal hygiene) and appearance (e.g., wearing face masks). These were individuals who tended to evaluate themselves in terms of how they thought they might appear to other people and then in terms of what other people might say about them (Earle et al., 2021).

Nudging and Adoption of Preventive Behaviours

Nudges have been used to encourage people to improve their personal hygiene practices. During the COVID-19 pandemic, regular handwashing and sanitisation, together with avoidance of face touching and the deep cleaning of surfaces in spaces frequently occupied or traversed by members of the public, were featured among the primary NPIs, enabling people to take some degree of personal control of their own protection from this infectious new disease. These "nudges" tended to comprise physical cues, which could be verbal and non-verbal, that pushed people subtly towards behaving in a specific way.

An example of the use of nudging in a handwashing context was the building of handwashing stations in school latrines in Bangladesh brightly decorated with handprints that reminded children of the need to wash their hands at these stations with messaging about making sure to use soap. These interventions were found to improve the incidence of handwashing in these schools from 4% to 68% the following day after their introduction and to 74% when further observations were taken two weeks and six weeks later (Dreibelbis et al., 2016; Grover et al., 2018). Nudge techniques have been found to produce outcomes every bit as successful as high-intensity health education programmes (Grover et al., 2018).

The establishment of nudge techniques across a range of health settings before the COVID-19 pandemic understandably reinforced pandemic control strategy (Rosenbaum, 2020). Nudging people to keep themselves and the spaces they spent time in cleaner was an obvious tool to recommend in the early days of the pandemic when there was still much to learn about it, including the eventual understanding that it was largely airborne.

Nudging encourages people to change their behaviour through subtle hints placed in their environment. There is no direct attempt to persuade people to change. Instead, when nudging methods are being deployed, people might be unaware of what is happening. Yet, very often they will respond to the "nudges" they encounter. "Boosting" is about equipping individuals with relevant data, information or knowledge about a behaviour and its advantages or disadvantages so that they can make more considered judgements about how to behave in future. In the hospital hygiene experiment, this comprised enhancements to hygiene literacy of the clinical staff.

In nudging, people make their own choices about how to behave but they often succumb to the subtle techniques being deployed to push their choices in the direction of a specific desired behaviour (Thaler & Sunstein, 2008). Critics have called out this technique as a form of libertarian paternalism (Hausman & Welch, 2010). Yet, its defenders would claim that it does not restrict people's choices; it simply pushes them towards a specific behavioural option (De Ridder et al., 2020).

Van Roekel et al. (2021) used "nudging" and "boosting" methods in a hospital setting to improve rates of good hand hygiene among medical and nursing staff. Over a four-week period, both methods were found to produce successful result compared to a control condition in which hospital staff received no intervention. The nudge approach produced a stronger immediate effect. The boost approach produced a more stable result over a longer time.

Nudges do not always work. They work best when they are deployed from a number of different directions such that people receive repeat hints about the behaviour to be changed (Frey & Rogers, 2014). In the hospital study reported above, the nudge technique was used to shift the mindset that medical and nursing staff had about hygiene from seeing it as an additional burden or chore on top of all their other concerns to a behaviour that protected patients. The boosting approach provided nurses with information about the extra risks to patients caused by poor hand hygiene on the part of staff, with factual statistical evidence about the likely rise in infections with poor hand hygiene. The nudging approach produced the stronger immediate effect on the target behaviour. When the interventions were taken away again, however, it was the group in the boosting condition that exhibited the most sustained behaviour change.

Nudging can be achieved through environmental cues and signs, but also via messaging that presents cost-benefit analyses of outcomes and spells out risks associated with specific behaviours. Adoption of behaviours as new habits, however, could be further motivated by risk perceptions and knowledge of specific interventions and the protection they can potentially provide (Dai et al., 2020; King et al., 2016; Mitchell et al., 2011; Park et al., 2010; Wise et al., 2020).

Group Processes and Self-Identity Model

Research undertaken before the COVID-19 pandemic indicated that although some personal hygiene measures were very widely adopted in many populations, others were much less so. In many instances, adoption levels for hand hygiene in terms of people following these practices most of the time average below half the population (Cowling et al., 2010; Salman et al., 2020).

In some cases, there were regional differences in compliance underpinned by a preponderance of specific cultural groups in an area that did not want to follow the restrictions. Often, there were political and religious reasons at play driving these cultural differences. There were differences between individuals in their perceptions of risk in terms of their own susceptibility and also in levels of fear of COVID-19 (Plohl & Musil, 2020).

Other situational factors could also come into play to influence propensity to comply with pandemic-related restrictions on their behaviour. There were variances in acceptance of and compliance with these rules that were linked to ethnicity, education, income, interpersonal relationships, structure of family household, and the kind of community in which people lived (Bradley et al., 2020). These kinds of variances in public compliance with rules cascaded down to them from authorities had been known about for some time (McLeroy et al., 1988).

The social ecological model examined a range of such societal and community level factors that could play significant roles in shaping public behaviour. It was helpful in identifying the kinds of public behaviour change interventions that would be most likely to achieve success within specific. It could be important to known about these mediating variables, especially in relation to women who often take pole position in taking health-related decisions for their families (Chen et al., 2018; Niermann et al., 2018; Nourijelyani et al., 2014; Waite & Gallagher, 2001).

The concept of trust also featured prominently in relation to the public's willingness to adopt behavioural interventions during pandemics and this applied to personal hygiene measures and social distancing. In this instance, people needed to trust the message(s) being received about behaviour change and most especially they needed to trust to source (of the message(s)). So, as well as developing a positive attitude towards social distancing in light of risk calculations, and then having established that others were observing these behavioural practices (social norms) and that they were capable of doing so themselves (behavioural control), people needed to have faith that the sources encouraging to adopt these new behaviours could be trusted (Gaygisiz et al., 2012; Liao et al., 2010).

Research by the WHO Europe (2020) reported that public trust in government policies associated with pandemic-related interventions was statistically associated with perceptions of the fairness of policies. The adoption of personal protection measures and social distancing behaviour was related to the efficacy of such measures when properly applied. If a person believed they could adopt these measures sufficiently to get genuine protection from them, then they were more likely to do so.

In a further analysis of the adoption of COVID-19-related preventive behaviours in different countries, Fujii et al. (2021) surveyed adult (18+) samples in China, Italy, Japan, Korea, the United Kingdom and the United States. The study focused on three protective behaviours: wearing a face mask, handwashing and avoidance of social gatherings. Adoption of these behaviours in virtually every country surveyed was more likely to occur among those who perceived that these behaviours were effective in controlling the spread of the coronavirus. There were some countries, however, in which adoption of preventive behaviours was not significantly linked to personal perceptions of their effectiveness in controlling the pandemic. The recommendations of medical experts and public health officials influenced people's decisions to take greater care through adoption of these protective behaviours. This outcome might also have meant that these sources were trusted by people in those locations.

In spite of the previous findings, self-efficacy was confirmed elsewhere as an important mediating variable in relation to adoption of social distancing behaviours (Liao et al., 2010). Combined with this variable were trust in the message and source, attitudes that represented positive feelings about social distancing, the perceived effectiveness of these behaviours and risk perceptions. Although support for each of these measures has not emerged as statistically significant in all studies that have tested them, there has been sufficient empirical evidence in each case to conclude that none should be ignored in models attempting to explain the adoption of social distancing behaviours during pandemics.

As we can see, compliance with public health measures such as those deployed during the 2020–2021 coronavirus pandemic can be influenced by group dynamics. This means that people often turn to specific social groups to which they belong or with which they identify for a steer in terms of how they should behave. Different membership or reference group allegiances can pull people in different directions over compliance with pandemic-related behavioural restrictions. Further research showed that as well as these judgements being influenced by pre-existing social groups, new groups emerged during the pandemic that were defined by positions adopted by different sectors of a population in regard to pandemic-related restrictions. One study of this phenomenon in the United Kingdom revealed two groups that emerged defined by their trust in science. One group exhibited trust in experts and the other did not. These groups not only diverged in terms of these alliances but also in their reported behaviour (Maher et al., 2020).

In another interesting demonstration of the new social "tribes" that emerged during the pandemic based upon people's orientations towards specific pandemic-related protection or control behaviours, American researchers found that face mask wearers and non-wearers differed in terms of how they reacted to others whose mask-wearing behaviour did or did not comply with their own. For instance, in an experiment that invited those taking part to cooperate with each other on specific tasks, non-mask wearers were significantly less likely to cooperate with a known mask wearer than with another known non-mask wearer (Powdthavee et al., 2021).

It was already known that there was a "tribal" divide in orientation towards wearing face masks based on established political allegiances. Political conservatives in the United States were less likely than liberals to wear face masks (Faciani, 2020). This division in behaviour was confirmed in studies comparing the views of Democrat and Republican voters (Rojas, 2020; Yeung et al., 2020). One reason for this difference was that Democrat supporters perceived greater risk from COVID-19 than did Republicans and hence were more willing to embrace protective measures such as face mask wearing (de Bruin et al., 2020).

Hence, the propensity to adopt protective behavioural measures against COVID-19 was linked to social perceptions and social identity. In the examples discussed, the political identity of individuals, which forms part of their wider self- or social-identity, was found to be an important mediating variable that determined how different people responded to the pandemic (Huddy & Bankert, 2017). If a behaviour such as mask wearing is associated with a specific social group and is known to be eschewed by another, members of the latter might be less inclined to wear masks despite nevertheless experiencing risk and related fear of infection. The pressure on them to conform to the behaviour of their reference group could outweigh the need for self-protection (Bohnet et al., 2008). Their reluctance to be disloyal to their tribe means they might even fail to take recommended steps to protect themselves even though they might fall into an "at risk" group as defined by their health status (Tang et al., 2017).

Theory of Planned Behaviour and Adoption of Preventive Behaviours

The public's knowledge and understanding of COVID-19 has also emerged as an important factor to increase the likelihood or adoption of preventive behaviours. Better knowledge can encourage more positive attitudes towards these behaviours and enhance the development that their adoption is in the wider public interest and will be endorsed by many people (Ammar et al., 2020; Andarge et al., 2020; Han et al., 2020; Prasetyo et al., 2020). Overall, though, perceived behavioural control regularly emerges as the most powerful predictor of behaviour.

Pre-COVID-19 pandemic research indicated that concepts from the theory of planned behaviour can predict adoption of personal hygiene measures. Regular handwashing tended to be performed by those already accustomed to doing so. It was also influenced by how busy people were and whether they "had the time" to perform this behaviour diligently. This behaviour might be regarded as being underpinned a subjective judgement of behaviour control, that is, the perception by the individual that they are able to do it or not. Surface cleaning was related to whether individuals had a regular cleaning routine, whether they thought that specific surfaces were dirty, and also whether they thought other people were being diligent about this. In theory of planned behaviour terms, therefore, the subjective norms predictor surfaced as an important precursor of target behaviour (Aunger et al., 2016).

A study of 3,693 Chinese students investigated their intentions to perform preventive behaviours associated with COVID-19 and the variables that could predict these intentions. Theory of planned behaviour constructs was included among the hypothesised predictor variables along with institutional climate of their university towards the pandemic and perceived risk of COVID-19. The institution's attitude towards the pandemic was an important orienting factor and theory of planned behaviour (TPB) variables such as attitude towards preventive behaviour, subjective norm and perceived behavioural control also had significant, though weaker impacts. Perceived risks of COVID-19 also further enhanced the impact of TPB variables (Li et al., 2021).

Research conducted in the United States found that perceived behavioural control, attitudes and subjective norm were all predictors of adoption of specific preventive behaviours, such as washing hands, using hand sanitiser, not touching your face, social distancing, wearing a face mask, disinfecting surfaces, coughing into your elbow and staying home when symptomatic. Behaviour control was an especially important predictor of adoption of preventive behaviour among older people. Subjective norm predicted all preventive behaviours except coughing into your elbow. Internalised attitudes towards social distancing were better predictors of social distancing than was perceived behavioural control (Aschwanden et al., 2021).

These results showed that internalised beliefs and attitudes are important antecedents of behaviour. Many of the preventive behaviours associated with COVID-19 were predicted by these psychological variables. Hence, knowing where people stand on using these behaviours and how they perceive the behaviours or others can help those trying to control public behaviour to develop messages to do the job.

Adherence to behavioural measures among adolescents in South Korea, as infection rates were increasing in that age group, was seen as critical to bringing the pandemic under control. A study that used the theory of planned behaviour to frame its inquiry considered whether adolescents' attitude and beliefs concerning COVID-related restrictions, their perceptions of how other were behaving and their personal abilities to comply with restrictions predicted intentions to comply (Park & Oh, 2021).

A face-to-face survey with 272 young people found that, in general, Korean adolescents were more inclined to comply with advisories such as wearing face masks than with physical distancing measures. The inclination to comply with COVID-linked restrictions was also statistically associated with perceptions of their personal susceptibility to catch the disease and of how severely ill this would make them, and with their perceptions of others' behaviours and with how difficult for themselves they thought compliance would be. These perceptions coupled with the subsequent strength of their intention to comply explained over 61% of the variance in their eventual reported behaviour. The researchers concluded that education targeted at this age group that promoted relevant beliefs and perceptions was important to procuring the eventual desired behavioural outcomes among young people.

In Pakistan, the theory of planned behaviour underpinned the design of a study of persuading people to wear face masks. There were particularly three important variables at play in this setting. These comprised the perceived risks from COVID-19, the perceived benefits of face masks, and the availability of face masks (or more to the point, their unavailability). These factors and perceived social norms concerning the wearing of face masks predicted the intention to wear face masks.

The findings here were interpreted as showing that public health authorities could play on public risk perceptions about COVID-19, but what was perhaps even more important was that people needed to perceive them to have relevant protective benefits and they had to be available for an affordable price. Lack of availability would mean that people in Pakistan would have little control over this behaviour and would therefore not be able to comply with it even if they wanted to (Irfan et al., 2021).

Another international study conducted via an online questionnaire survey covered participants from six countries, China, Japan and South Korea in the east and Italy, the United Kingdom and the United States in the west. Willingness to take protective behavioural measures such as wearing face masks, regular handwashing and keeping your distance from other people were more likely to be reported as being adopted by people who believed these measures could offer real and effective protection (Fujii et al., 2021).

COM-B Approach

Moving beyond these models, other psychologists have identified additional variables and combinations of variables that might make a difference to whether people will comply with restrictions imposed from above on their behaviour. The nudge and planned behaviour models, as we have seen, have produced positive results from studies that have demonstrated that they have some explanatory efficacy in relation to pandemic behaviour restrictions and adoption of protective behaviours. These models, however, tend to confine their theorising around specific sets of factors. A widespread scan of psychological research, however, can reveal other predictors of this behaviour. Indeed, there could be benefits for understanding to be gained from sometimes combining predictor variables from nudge theory and planned behaviour theory and then also from other theories.

While having theory is important in any research to provide explanation of relationships between variables and then to be able to forecast an event's consequences or outcomes, single theoretical models might be too narrowly definitive of key variables and choices in the context of major crises. In the case of pandemics, and especially one that affected the entire world on the scale of COVID-19, some experts have advised that a wider approach might be advisable in trying to understanding how to tackle such events (Bish & Michie, 2010). By taking this approach, evidence will be considered from a broader pool of research.

In effect, Bish and Michie were recommending the integration of different models that had previously been found to offer some relevance to the systematic of pandemics. Where a large-scale event necessitated extensive and diverse public behaviour changes, achievement of this outcome was likely to depend upon the application of a wide range of interventions. Not only did each of these interventions need to be effective in producing a specific change to people's behaviour patterns (e.g., making a point of keeping physically apart), when more than one intervention was used in combination with others, there needed to be some certainty that they would work effectively together. The last thing anyone would want if that the impact of one intervention counteracts or neutralises the impact of another.

When Bish and Michie (2010) were examining research that was underpinned by theory in the health sphere, they found that relatively few studies were theoretically grounded. When they were, there were two models that were utilised most often: the health belief model and the theory of planned behaviour. Other theories also surfaced in specific studies. Kupfer and colleagues studied the factors that motivated the practice of good hand hygiene using the theory of interpersonal behaviour (Kupfer et al., 2020).

On examining research from earlier pandemics, Bish and Michie found that different researchers identified many different psychological variables that could have shaped public behaviour. Sometimes, pandemic-related behaviour was influenced by risk perceptions which would include perceived risks to self and others and severity of disease once infected. Other studies examined whether people felt able to take protective steps and whether these steps were regarded as effective in the protection they could provide (King et al., 2016; Mitchell et al., 2011; Park et al., 2010; Rubin et al., 2009). Other variables of importance included demographic measures such as age, gender and ethnicity (Kamate et al., 2009; Kim & Niederdeppe, 2013).

There is plentiful evidence that public knowledge and understanding of protective behaviours is important to their adoption by a population. In the COVID-19 pandemic research across a range of populations showed that large majorities increased their handwashing behaviour after being told that this could offer them some protection (Mitchell et al., 2011; Rubin et al., 2009; Salman et al., 2020; Taghrir et al., 2020).

Review of further evidence indicated that although some hygiene measures were very widely adopted in many populations, others were much less so. In many instances, adoption levels for hand hygiene in terms of people following these practices most or all of the time average below half the population (Liao et al., 2010; Cowling et al., 2010; Salman et al., 2020).

Some psychologists devoted attention to establishing whether the propensity of people to comply with preventive behaviours had its own distinctive psychometric properties. One group developed a scale called the COVID-19 Preventive Behaviours Index (CPBI) with this aim in mind. Other psychological scales that emerged during the pandemic included the Fear of COVID-19 Scale and the COVID-19 Own Risk Appraisal Scale, both of which were found to yield scores about test samples that correlated highly with scores on the CPBI (Breakwell et al., 2021). Hence, relevant psychological tests indicated that greater fear of COVID-19 and high personal risk perceptions were strongly associated with greater propensities to adopt preventive behaviours.

Changing behaviour also usually requires earlier changes to internal psychological constructs such as attitudes, beliefs, perceptions and motivations. They might also depend upon knowledge changes and internalised risk assessments. All of these shifts of psychological drivers of behaviour must occur in a timely way and must work in harmony together. People must want to change their behaviour, must believe that the benefits of such behaviour change outweigh any costs, must feel good about making this change, must perceive that such behaviour change is expected by other people (especially those who represent important reference points or role models), and must believe they are capable of making this change. If a multitude of behaviour changes are required at the same time or within a fairly brief window of time, this can place a considerable psychological load on them (Aunger et al., 2016).

Knowledge of various NPIs that can be adopted by individuals such as hand hygiene and social distancing is a precursor to motivation to comply. People must understand how to use these measures and why they are important, as well as how effective they can be. This awareness also requires some degree of understanding of the disease from which they are being protected and its mode(s) of transmission.

There was pandemic-related evidence gathered in 2020 that public knowledge and understanding of protective behaviours is important to their adoption by a population. In the COVID-19 pandemic research across a range of populations showed that large majorities increased their hand-washing behaviour after being told that this could offer them some protection (Salman et al., 2020; Taghrir et al., 2020).

Linked to this knowledge are risk perceptions that comprise calculations made by individuals about their own chances of becoming infected. Those who perceive themselves to be more at risk will tend to be more strongly motivated to adopted protective measures. Risks will in effect "nudge" people towards changing their behaviour. Knowledge does not guarantee adoption of behaviour because the behaviour itself must be perceived as being within the scope of the individual. This involves a rational judgement as indicated by notion of "planned behaviour" and could weaken or magnify the effects of the "nudge".

Hence the I-change model proposed by Bish and Michie (2010) offered more flexibility by embracing different constructs from different models rather than by attaching itself to only model that might not offer a sufficient range of explanatory concepts to comprehensively account for any behaviour change that is achieved.

With hand hygiene and other personal protective behaviours, explanations were needed that would draw from all relevant theoretical models and studies that demonstrated their explanatory efficacy. Various factor types also needed to be differentiated. There were predisposing factors that created the conditions for internal motivations or intentions to behave to emerge. Then internal intentions needed to be connected theoretically and empirically to actual behavioural outcomes. Predisposing factors might include demographics and psychological classifiers (personality attributes), knowledge, prior experiences and knowledge. In the case of handwashing, for instance, there might also have been a pre-established habit factor defined by pre-pandemic diligence on the part of some individuals to wash their hands regularly.

The COM-B model was judged to provide a number of useful indications for future policy. With hygiene practices, it was recommended that government and public health messaging should reinforce public motivation to persist with these behaviours and to internalise the reasons why it was generally good health practice. Some population sub-groups would need closer attention than others to encourage them to persist with these behaviours. Men, for example, appeared to need more encouragement than women and younger people more than older people (Gibson-Miller et al., 2021).

Lessons Learned

Personal protective measures such as handwashing, good coughing hygiene and wearing of face coverings have been found to represent important interventions that can reduce the spread of infectious viruses such as SARS-CoV-2. They cannot totally control the spread of diseases that are also airborne, but they can form effective components of a multi-faceted pandemic control strategy. Some countries, most notably in Asia, had already adopted face mask wearing as a normative behaviour before the novel coronavirus pandemic. This was not the case in many other parts of the world. Socialising people to adopt new behaviours such as these is achievable but is not always easy. There will always be a few people who will refuse to comply.

The evidence presented in this chapter showed that the four psychological models being examined in this book had each been deployed in the context of encouraging populations to adopt personal protective behaviours. Establishing such behaviours could be achieved through appropriate environmental cues, through references to the behaviour of others, through cognitive reasoning and by creating relevant motivational states. Ultimately, individuals must be willing to adopt these practices. Forcing them on people might result in psychological reactance with some population sub-groups refusing to comply on principle. Getting the right messages across about adoption of these measures is critical to minimise resistance. Measures such as good hygiene and face mask wearing had been shown provide effective barriers to the spread of COVID-19 (Talic, 2021). To work effectively, they need to be adopted by most people and people must be willing to engage with necessary protective behaviour, knowing that they can do this and knowing the benefits it will bring.

References

Allcott, H., Boxell, L., Conway, J., Gentzkow, M., Thaler, M., & Yang, D. Y. (2020). Polarization and public health: Partisan differences in social distancing during the coronavirus pandemic. *NBER Working Paper 2020* (w26946). Available online: https://ssrn.com/abstract=3574415

Ammar, N., Aly, N. M., Folayan, M. O., Khader, Y., Virtanen, J. I., Al-Batayneh, O. B., et al. (2020). Behavior change due to COVID-19 among dental academics – the theory of planned behaviour: stresses, worries, training, and pandemic severity. *PLoS One, 15*, e0239961. https://doi.org/10.1371/journal.pone.0239961

Andarge, E., Fikadu, T., Temesgen, R., Shegaze, M., Feleke, T., Haile, F., et al. (2020). Intention and practice on personal preventive measures against the covid-19 pandemic among adults with chronic conditions in southern Ethiopia: A survey using the theory of planned behaviour. *Journal of Multidisciplinary Healthcare, 13*, 1863–1877. https://doi.org/10.2147/JMDH.S284707

Anderson, K. M., & Stockmarr, J. K. (2021). Staying home, distancing and face masks: COVID-19 prevention among U.S. women in the COPE study. *International Journal of Environmental Research and Public Health, 18*(1), 180. https://doi.org/10.3390/ijerph18010180

Aschwanden, D., Strickhouser, J. E., Sesker, A. A., Lee, J. H., Luchetti, M., Terracciano, A., & Sutin, A. R. (2021). Preventive behaviors during the COVID-19 pandemic: Associations with perceived behavioral control, attitudes, and subjective norms. *Frontiers in Public Health, 9*, 662835. https://doi.org/10.3389/fpubh.2021.662835

Aunger, R., Greenland, K., Ploubidis, G., Schmidt, W., Oxford, J., & Curtis, V. (2016). The determinants of reported personal and household hygiene behaviour: A multi-country study. *PLoS One, 11*(8), e0159551. Retrieved from: https://journals.plos.org/plosone/article?id=10.1371/journal.pone.0159551

Berg, M. B., & Lin, L. (2020). Prevalence and predictors of early COVID-19 behavioral intentions in the United States. *Translational Behavioural Medicine, 10*, 843–849.

Berkman, N. D., Sheridan, S. L., Donahue, K. E., Halpern, D. J., & Crotty, K. (2011). Low health literacy and health outcomes: An updated systematic review. *Annals of Internal Medicine, 155*, 97–107.

Bish, A., & Michie, S. (2010). Demographic and attitudinal determinants of protective behaviours during a pandemic: A review. *British Journal of Health Psychology, 15*(4), 797–824.

Bohnet, I., Greig, F., Herrmann, B., & Zeckhauser, R. (2008). Betrayal aversion: Evidence from Brazil, China, Oman, Switzerland, Turkey, and the United States. *American Economic Review, 98*(1), 294–310.

Bradley, D. T., Mansouri, M. A., Kee, F., & Garcia, L. M. T. (2020). A systems approach to preventing and responding to COVID-19. *EClinicalMedicine, 21*, 100325.

Breakwell, G. M., Fino, E., & Jaspal, R. (2021). The COVID-19 Preventive Behaviors Index: Development and validation in two samples from the United Kingdom. *Evaluation & the Health Professions, 44*(1), 77–86. https://doi.org/10.1177/0163278720983416

Calogero, R. M., Tylka, T. L., Siegel, J. A., & Pina, A. (2020). Smile pretty and watch your back: Personal safety anxiety and vigilance to objectification theory. *Journal of Personality and Social Psychology*. https://doi.org/10.1037/pspi0000344.

Centers for Disease Control and Prevention Coronavirus Disease 2019: Racial & Ethnic Minority Groups. (2020). Available online: https://www.cdc.gov/coronavirus/2019-ncov/need-extra-precautions/racial-ethnic-minorities.html (accessed on 20 June 2020).

Chen, J.-L., Guo, J., Esquivel, J. H., & Chesla, C. A. (2018). Like mother, like child: The influences of maternal attitudes and behaviours on weight-related health behaviours in their children. *Journal of Transcultural Nursing, 29*, 523–531.

Chen, Y. J., Qin, G., Chen, J., Xu, J. L., Feng, D. Y., Wu, X. Y., & Li, X. (2020). Comparison of face-touching behaviours before and during the coronavirus disease 2019 pandemic. *JAMA Network Open, 3*(7), e2016924. https://doi.org/10.1001/jamanetworkopen.2020.16924

Chu, D. K., Akl, E. A., Duda, S., et al. (2020). Physical distancing, face masks, and eye protection to prevent person-to-person transmission of SARS-CoV-2 and COVID-19: A systematic review and meta-analysis. *Lancet, 395*, 1973–1987.

Cowling, B. J., Ali, S. T., Ng, T. W. Y., Tsang, T. K., Li, J. C. M., Fong, M. W., Liao, Q., Kwan, M. Y. W., Lee, S. L., Chiu, S. S., et al. (2020). Impact assessment of non-pharmaceutical interventions against coronavirus disease 2019 and influenza in Hong Kong: An observational study. *Lancet Public Health, 5*, e279–e288.

Cowling, B. J., Ng, D. M., Ip, D. K., Liao, Q., Lam, W. W., Wu, J. T., Lau, J. T., Griffiths, S. M., & Fielding, R. (2010). Community psychological and behavioral responses through the first wave of the 2009 influenza A (H1N1) pandemic in Hong Kong. *Journal of Infectious Diseases, 202*(6), 867–876. https://doi.org/10.1086/655811

Dai, B., Fu, D., Meng, G., Liu, B., Li, Q., & Liu, X. (2020). The effects of governmental and individual predictors on COVID-19 protective behaviors in China: A path analysis model. *Public Administration Review*. https://doi.org/10.1111/puar.13236

de Bruin, W. B., Saw, H. W., & Goldman, D. P. (2020). Political polarization in U.S. residents' COVID-19 risk perceptions, policy preferences, and protective behaviours. *Journal of Risk Uncertainty, 61*(2), 177–194.

De Ridder, D., Feitsma, J., Van den Hoven, M., Kroese, F., Schillemans, T., Verwell, M., & De Vet, E. (2020). Simple nudges that are not so easy. *Behavioural Public Policy*, 1–19. https://doi.org/10.1017/bpp.2020.36

Dreibelbis, R., Kroeger, A., & Ram, P. K. (2016). Behavior change without behaviour change communication: Nudging handwashing among primary school students in Bangladesh. *International Journal of Environmental Research and Public Health, 13*(1), 129. https://doi.org/10.3390/ijerph13010129

Earle, M., Prusaczyk, E., Choma, B., & Calogero, R. (2021). Compliance with COVID-19 safety measures: A test of an objectification theory model. *Body Image, 37*, 6–13.

Faciani, M. (2020, 9th September). How did mask wearing become so politicized? *The Conversation* [Cited 13 May 2021]. Available from: https://theconversation.com/video-how-did-mask-wearing-become-so-politicized-144268

Fitzpatrick, K. M., Harris, C., & Drawve, G. (2020). Fear of COVID-19 and the mental health consequences in America. *Psychological Trauma, 12*, S17–S21.

Frey, E., & Rogers, T. (2014). Persistence: How treatment effects persist after interventions stop. *Policy Insights from the Behavioural and Brain Sciences*, 1(1), 172–179.

Fujii, R., Suzuki, K., & Niimi, J. (2021). Public perceptions, individual characteristics, and preventive behaviors for COVID-19 in six countries: A cross-sectional study. *Environmental Health and Preventive Medicine*, 26(1), 29. https://doi.org/10.1186/s12199-021-00952-2

Gaygisiz, Ü., Gaygisiz, E., Özkan, T., & Lajunen, T. (2012). Individual differences in behavioral reactions to H1N1 during a later stage of the epidemic. *Journal of Infections and Public Health*, 5(1), 9–21.

Gibson-Miller, J., Zavlis, O., Hartman, T. K., McBride, O., Bennett, K., Butter, S., Levita, L., Mason, L., Martinez, A. P., McKay, R., Murphy, J., Shevlin, M., Stocks, T. V. A., & Bentall, R. P. (2021). Psychological factors influencing protective behaviours during the COVID-19 pandemic: Capability, opportunity and motivation. In F. Gabrielli & F. Irtelli (Eds.), *Anxiety, Uncertainty, and Resilience during the Pandemic Period – Anthropological and Psychological Perspectives* (online ahead of print). Intech Open. https://doi.org/10.5772/intechopen.98237

Grover, E., Hossain, M. K., Uddin, S., Venkatesh, M., Ram, P. K., & Dreibelbis, R. (2018). Comparing the behavioural impact of a nudge-based handwashing intervention to high-intensity hygiene education: A cluster-randomised trial in rural Bangladesh. *Tropical Medicine and International Health*, 23(1), 10–25.

Haffajee, R. L., & Mello, M. M. (2020). Thinking globally, acting locally – the US response to COVID-19. *New England Journal of Medicine*, 382(22), e75. https://doi.org/10.1026/NEJMp2006740

Han, H., Al-Ansi, A., Chua, B.-L., Tariq, B., Radic, A., & Park, S. (2020). The post-coronavirus world in the international tourism industry: Application of the theory of planned behavior to safer destination choices in the case of us outbound tourism. *International Journal of Environmental Research and Public Health*, 17, 6485. https://doi.org/10.3390/ijerph17186485

Harper, C. A., Satchell, L. P., Fido, D., & Latzman, R. D. (2020). Functional fear predicts public health compliance in the COVID-19 pandemic. *International Journal of Mental Health and Addiction*, 1–14 [Epublication ahead of print]. https://doi.org/10.1007/s11469-020-00281-5

Hausman, D. M., & Welch, B. (2010). Debate: To nudge or not to nudge. *Journal of Political Philosophy*, 18(1), 123–136

Howard, J., Huang, A., Li, Z., Tufekci, Z., Zdimal, V., van der Westhuizen, H. M., von Delft, A., Price, A., Fridman, L., Tang, L. H., Tang, V., Watson, G. L., Bax, C. E., Shaikh, R., Questier, F., Hernandez, D., Chu, L. F., Ramirez, C. M., & Rimoin, A. W. (2021). An evidence review of face masks against COVID-19. *Proceedings of the National Academy of Science USA*, 118(4), e2014564118. https://doi.org/10.1073/pnas.2014564118

Huddy, L., & Bankert, A. (2017). Political partisanship as a social identity. In *Oxford Research Encyclopedias of Politics*. https://doi.org/10.1093/acrefore/9780190228637.013.250

Irfan, M., Akhtar, N., Ahmad, M., Shahzad, F., Elavarasan, R. M., Wu, H., & Yang, C. (2021). Assessing public willingness to wear face masks during the COVID-19 pandemic: Fresh insights from the theory of planned behaviour. *International Journal of Environmental Research and Public Health, 18*(9), 4577. https://doi.org/10.3390/ijerph18094577

Kamate, S. K., Agrawal, A., Chaudhary, H., Singh, K., Mishra, P., Asawa, K. (2009). Public knowledge, attitude and behavioural changes in an Indian population during the Influenza A (H1N1) outbreak. *Journal of Infection in Developing Countries, 4*(1), 7–14. https://doi.org/10.3855/jidc.501

Kantamneni, N. (2020). The impact of the COVID-19 pandemic on marginalized populations in the United States: A research agenda. *Journal of Vocational Behaviour, 119*, 103439.

Kim, H. K., & Niederdeppe, J. (2013). Exploring optimistic bias and the integrative model of behavioural prediction in the context of a campus influenza outbreak. *Journal of Health Communication, 18*(2), 206–222.

King, D. B., Kamble, S., & DeLongis, A. (2016). Coping with influenza A/H1N1 in India: Empathy is associated with increased vaccination and health precautions. *International Journal of Health Promotion and Education, 54*(6), 283–294.

Kupfer, T. R., Wyles, K. J., Watson, F., La Ragione, R. M., Chambers, M. A., & Macdonald, A. S. (2020). Determinants of hand hygiene behaviour based on the theory of interpersonal behaviour. *Journal of Infection Prevention, 20*(5), 232–237.

Li, J., Liu, X., Zou, Y., Deng, Y., Zhang, M., Yu, M., Wu, D., Zheng, H., & Zhao, X. (2021). Factors affecting COVID-19 preventive behaviours among university students in Beijing, China: An empirical study based on the Extended Theory of Planned Behaviour. *International Journal of Environmental Research and Public Health, 18*(13), 7009. https://doi.org/10.3390/ijerph18137009

Li, T., Liu, Y., Li, M., Qian, X., & Dai, S. Y. (2020). Mask or no mask for COVID-19: A public health and market study. *PLoS One, 15*(8), e0237691. https://doi.org/10.1371/journal.pone.0237691

Liao, Q., Cowling, B., Lam, W. T., Ng, M. W., & Fielding, R. (2010). Situational awareness and health protective responses to pandemic influenza A (H1N1) in Hong Kong: A cross-sectional study. *PLoS One, 5*(10), e13350.

Liu, X., & Zhang, S. (2020). COVID-19: Face masks and human-to-human transmission. *Influenza and Other Respiratory Viruses, 14*, 472–473.

Maher, P. J., MacCarron, P., & Quayle, M. (2020). Mapping public health responses with attitude networks: The emergence of opinion-based groups in the UK's early COVID-19 response phase. *British Journal of Social Psychology, 59*(3), 641–652. https://doi.org/10.1111/bjso.12396

McLeroy, K. R., Bibeau, D., Steckler, A., & Glanz, K. (1988). An ecological perspective on health promotion programs. *Health Education Quarterly, 15*, 51–377.

Mitchell, T., Dee, D. L., Phares, C. R., Lipman, H. B., Gould, L. H., Kutty, P., et al. (2011). Non-pharmaceutical interventions during an outbreak of 2009 pandemic influenza A (H1N1) virus infection at a large public university, April-May 2009. *Clinical Infectious Diseases, 52*(Suppl. 1), S138–S145.

Ngonghala, C. N., Iboi, E. A., & Gumel, A. B. (2020). Could masks curtail the post-lockdown resurgence of COVID-19 in the US? *Mathematical Biosciences, 329*, Article 108452. https://doi.org/10.1016/j.mbs.2020.108452

Niermann, C. Y. N., Spengler, S., & Gubbels, J. S. (2018). Physical activity, screen time, and dietary intake in families: A cluster-analysis with mother-father-child triads. *Frontiers in Public Health, 6*, 276. https://doi.org/10.3389/fpubh.2018.00276

Nourijelyani, K., Yekaninejad, M. S., Eshraghian, M., Mohammad, K., Foroushani, A. R., & Pakpour, A. (2014). The influence of mothers' lifestyle and health behaviour on their children: An exploration for oral health. *Iranian Red Crescent Medical Journal, 16*, e16051.

Park, J. H., Cheong, H. K., Son, D. Y., Kim, S. U., & Ha, C. M. (2010). Perceptions and behaviours related to hand hygiene for the prevention of H1N1 influenza transmission among Korean university students during the peak pandemic period. *BMC Infectious Diseases, 10*(1), 222.

Park, S., & Oh, S. (2021). Factors associated with preventive behaviours for COVID-19 among adolescents in South Korea. *Journal of Pediatric Nursing*, 10:S0882-5963(21)00210-4. https://doi.org/10.1016/j.pedn.2021.07.006

Plohl, N., & Musil, B. (2020). Modelling compliance with COVID-19 prevention guidelines: The critical role of trust in science. *Psychology, Health and Medicine, 26*(1), 1–12.

Poteat, T., Millett, G. A., Nelson, L. E., & Beyrer, C. (2020). Understanding COVID-19 risks and vulnerabilities among black communities in America: The lethal force of syndemics. *Annals of Epidemiology, 47*, 1–3.

Powdthavee, N., Riyanto, Y. E., Wong, E. C. L., Yeo, J. X. W., & Chan, Q. Y. (2021). When face masks signal social identity: Explaining the deep face-mask divide during the COVID-19 pandemic. *PLoS One, 16*(6), e0253195. https://doi.org/10.1371/journal.pone.0253195

Prasetyo, Y. T., Castillo, A. M., Salonga, L. J., Sia, J. A. & Seneta, J. A. (2020). Factors affecting perceived effectiveness of COVID-19 prevention measures among Filipinos during enhanced community quarantine in Luzon, Philippines: Integrating Protection Motivation Theory and extended Theory of Planned Behaviour. *International Journal of Infectious Diseases, 99*, 312–323. https://doi.org/10.1016/j.ijid.2020.07.074

Razzaghi, H., Wang, Y., Lu, H., Marshall, K. E., Dowling, N. F., Paz-Bailey, G., Twentyman, E. R., Peacock, G., & Greenlund, K. J. (2020). Estimated county-level prevalence of selected underlying medical conditions associated with increased risk for severe COVID-19 illness – United States, 2018. *MMWR Morbidity and Mortality Weekly Report, 69*, 945–950.

Rojas, R. (2020). Masks become a flashpoint in the virus culture wars. *The New York Times* [Cited 13 May 2021]. Available from: https://www.nytimes.com/2020/05/03/us/coronavirus-masks-protests.html

Rosenbaum, J. (2020, 31st March). Incorporating nudges into COVID-19 communication and prevention strategies. *Global Handwashing Partnership*. www.globalhandwashing.org/incorporating-nudges-into-covid-19-communication-and-prevention-strategies

Rubin, G. J., Amlôt, R., Page, L., & Wessely, S. (2009). Public perceptions, anxiety, and behaviour change in relation to the swine flu outbreak: Cross sectional telephone survey. *British Medical Journal, 339*(7713), 156.

Salman, M., Mustafa, Z. U., Asif, N., Zaidi, H. A., Hussain, K., Shehzadi, N., et al. (2020). Knowledge, attitude and preventive practices related to COVID-19: A cross-sectional study in two Pakistani university populations. *Drugs & Therapy Perspectives, 36*(7), 319–325.

Seale, H., Heywood, A. E., Leask, J., Sheel, M., Thomas, S., Durrheim, D. N., et al. (2020). COVID-19 is rapidly changing: Examining public perceptions and behaviours in response to this evolving pandemic. *PloS One, 15*, 6.

Song, L. J., Xu, S., Xu, S. L., Sun, Z., & Liu, W. (2020). Psychology of wearing face masks to prevent transition of COVID-19. *BMJ General Psychiatry, 23*(6). https://doi.org/10/1136/gpsych-2020-100297

Taghrir, M. H., Borazjani, R., & Shiraly, R. (2020). COVID-19 and Iranian medical students; a survey on their related-knowledge, preventive behaviours and risk perception. *Archives of Iranian Medicine, 23*(4), 249–254.

Talic, S. (2021). Effectiveness of public health measures in reducing the incidence of covid-19, SARS-CoV-2 transmission, and covid-19 mortality: Systematic review and meta-analysis. *Thebmj, 375*, e068302. Retrieved from: https://www.bmj.com/content/375/bmj-2021-068302

Tang, S., Morewedge, C. K., Larrick, R. P., & Klein, J. G. (2017). Disloyalty aversion: Greater reluctance to bet against close others than the self. *Organisational Behaviour and Human Decision Processes, 140*, 1–13.

Tannenbaum, M. B., Hepler, J., Zimmerman, R. S., Saul, L., Jacobs, S., Wilson, K., & Albarracin, D. (2015). Appeal to fear: A meta-analysis of fear appeal effectiveness and theories. *Psychological Bulletin, 141*, 1178–1204.

Thaler, R. H., & Sunstein, C. R. (2008). *Nudge: Improving Decisions about Health, Wealth and Happiness*. New Haven, Conn: Yale University Press.

Van Roekel, H., Reinhard, J., & Grimmelikhuijsen, S. (2021). Improving hand hygiene in hospitals: Comparing the effect of a nudge and a boost on protocol compliance. *Behavioural Public Policy*, 1–23. https://doi.org/10.1017/bpp.2021.15

Waite, L. J., & Gallagher, M. (2001). *The Case for Marriage: Why Married People Are Happier, Healthier, and Better Off Financially*. New York, NY: Random House Digital, Inc.

West, R., Michie, S., Rubin, G. J., & Amlot, R. (2020). Applying principles of behaviour change to reduce SARS-CoV-2 transmission .*Nature and Human Behaviour, 4*, 451–459.

WHO Europe. (2020). Survey tool and guidance. Rapid, simple, flexible behavioural insights on COVID-19. http://www.euro.who.int/__data/assets/pdf_file/0007/436705/COVID-19-survey-tool-and-guidance.pdf?ua=1 (accessed 14 April 2020).

Wise, T., Zbozinak, T., Michelini, G., Hagan, C., & Mobbs, D. (2020). Changes in risk perception and self-reported protective behaviour during the first week of the COVID-19 pandemic in the United States. *Royal Society Open Science, 7*, 200742.

World Health Organization. (2020). Advice on the use of masks in the context of COVID-19, interim guidance. Available: https://apps.who.int/iris/bitstream/handle/10665/332293/WHO-2019-nCov-IPC_Masks-2020.4-eng.pdf?sequence=1&isAllowed=y (accessed 20 July 2020).

Xu, H., Gan, Y., Zheng, D., Wu, B., Zhu, X., Xu, C., Liu, C., Tao, Z., Hu, Y., Chen, M., Li, M., Lu Z., & Chen, J. (2020). Relationship between COVID-19 infection and risk perception, knowledge, attitude, and four nonpharmaceutical interventions during the late period of the COVID-19 epidemic in China: Online cross-sectional survey of 8158 adults. *Journal of Medical and Internet Research*, 22(11), e21372. https://doi.org/10.2196/21372

Yeung, N., Lai, J., & Luo, J. (2020). Face off: Polarized public opinions on personal face mask usage during the COVID-19 pandemic. *arXiv* [Preprint arXiv:2011.00336]. Available from: https://arxiv.org/abs/2011.00336

Chapter 11

Return to Normality: The Public and Vaccination

During the early phases of large-scale non-pharmaceutical interventions (NPIs) designed to slow the spread of the new coronavirus – SARS-CoV-2 – publics around the world were told by their governments that their normal lives would need to be put on hold and restrictions on their behaviour might have to continue until a vaccine became available. Governments invested huge amounts of money in vaccine research in the hope of accelerating its development. Any approved vaccine would need to go through all the necessary trials to ensure that it worked by triggering the production of antibodies in humans that would fight off the virus and that it did not cause dangerous side effects. The crisis context in which this initiative occurred, however, meant that there was much greater urgency to get the job down than the usual timeframes for such scientific developments.

Yet, despite the advice of medical and scientific leaders that vaccination is ultimately the principal way out of the pandemic, significant numbers of people voiced concerns that the new vaccines might be unsafe or had some hidden agenda ultimately designed to enhance some centralised agencies' control over public behaviour beyond the pandemic, either for political purposes or financial gain. Others expressed concerns that the new vaccines had been developed so quickly, and certainly much faster than it usually takes, that they might not be safe. Hence, despite the promise that vaccines represented the ultimate rescue package, significant minorities threatened to refuse to be immunised.

There was evidence that those who had been infected by the coronavirus develop their own protection against further infection by developing antibodies and T-cells to neutralise the virus. What was not known by the end of 2020 was how long this protection would last. Evidence from other types of coronavirus infection had indicated that antibody responses could be short-lived (Edridge et al., 2020). Cases of reinfection by COVID-19 had been observed, but these numbered just a handful out of millions of known cases (Iwasaki, 2020). Hence there was considerable uncertainty about the longevity of naturally acquired protection against this disease. Vaccination could therefore provide a much-needed booster to the body's

DOI: 10.4324/9781003274308-11

immune system in a way relevant to identifying the virus if exposed to it again in the future. What would remain uncertain until vaccination programmes had been rolled out and had time to allow data collection showing the nature of the protection they provided, there would continue to be uncertainties about the vaccines and also an ongoing need to deploy other interventions placing behavioural restrictions on people (Mahase, 2020; *The Lancet*, 2021).

International data collected between 17th November 2020 and 10th January 2021 showed the proportions of people from the 24 surveyed countries who said that they were likely to get vaccinated when a vaccine became available. The variance ranged from a high of 83% in Thailand saying they would get vaccinated to a low of 28% in Poland. The United Kingdom came second with 80% saying they would get vaccinated. This still meant that one in five did not commit to getting immunised. These broke down into just over one in ten (11%) who "did not know" what they would do at the time they were asked and just under one in ten (9%) who said they would not get vaccinated (Smith, 2021; YouGov, 2021, 12th January).

There were wide, country-to-country disparities in willingness to accept and use vaccines for protection for example in Europe between nations such as France (39%), Germany (51%), Italy (64%) and Denmark (70%). Meanwhile, in the United States where there was an active anti-vaxxer movement, fewer than half the public (47%) exhibited any enthusiasm for COVID vaccination. While nearly half of French respondents (48%) did *not* want to get vaccinated, only 9% said they were anti-vaccination as a general principle. In the United States, one in four people (26%) did not want to get vaccinated against COVID but only a few (6%) were signed-up anti-vaxxers. A more important consideration of those displaying vaccine hesitancy was whether the new vaccines were safe (Smith, 2021).

In the United Kingdom, the public's willingness to get vaccinated gradually evolved over time. When initially surveyed on this in November 2020, just over six in ten (61%) showed enthusiasm for COVID vaccination. By the beginning of 2021, as the vaccine roll-out got underway with those "most at risk", vaccine acceptance grew to eight in ten (80%). By the beginning of May 2021, this had grown still further to nine in ten (90%) (YouGov, 2021, 12th January; accessed 15th June 2021).

Vaccination Uptake

Getting the public on board with vaccination calls for more than scientific and safety assurances. Historically, public opposition to or at least caution about vaccination programmes was grounded in people's perceptions of authorities in health and politics that were pushing for this solution to public health issues to be adopted. Experience has taught that it is important, indeed essential, to use narratives about new vaccines that show the good they can do in communities. Such messaging can go a long way towards cultivating and securing public confidence in such scientific developments (Harrison & Wu, 2020).

A further factor in play with vaccination programmes is the ideal of freedom of choice. In many developed societies around the world, people are accustomed to being permitted to make up their own minds about how they live their lives and about the choices they may make in relation to caring for their own health. Hence, being told by an authority that they must get vaccinated sits uncomfortably with this cultural ideal. If people believe they are being coerced into a behaviour, then even when they are told it is for their own good, they might be inclined to push back against it. The concept of "psychological reactance" is relevant in this context.

It is also worth remembering that with the implementation of many NPIs to restrict public behaviour, many people believed they were already being forced to abandon their normal lives and comply with rules they often regarded as unjust or unfair. Being confronted with another requirement on top of everything else might prove to be too much and reactance might therefore be more likely to occur against vaccination. In countering this resistance, authorities need to demonstrate to those whose behaviour they are seeking to influence that vaccination will have genuine personal and community-wide benefits (Harrison & Wu, 2020). The idea that others were starting to comply, if substantiated through their own experience, would also help to push resisters towards compliance with immunisation requests.

Nudging People Along

When campaigns are run that seek to influence the way people behave, their outcomes can depend upon the ways in which different arguments are presented and, in particular, the different choices that are offered to people. Ultimately, those receiving such messages must decide whether they want to change or not and whether they want to comply or not with the persuasive messages presented to them. The way campaigns and their messages are constructed has been referred to as *choice architecture* (Johnson & Goldstein, 2003; Scheibehenne et al., 2010). The choice architecture can vary the number of behaviour choices presented to people, the characteristics of each choice, and might also present one behaviour as a default, with other options people must deliberately opt into while opting out of the one given to them (Thaler et al., 2013).

With nudge approaches, the aim is to encourage people to make rational decisions with which they are comfortable and which, at the same time, result in behaviour changes that public health authorities or governments are seeking to achieve. The intention always is not to force people to change but to persuade them that a specific pattern of behaviour might be more advantageous for them under specific sets of circumstances. In this context, behaviour change occurs because people want it and not because it has been mandated by government or another authority. Mandating change, without giving people an opportunity to decide for themselves, can trigger reactance whereby people push back against or reject the change being forced upon them (Goodwin, 2016; Johnson et al., 2012).

Choice architecture can comprise a number of specific elements that might be used individually or together. Among the tools of the trade are the uses of defaults whereby a specific behaviour is offered up to people as the one they will be automatically signed up to unless they stipulate otherwise. Under such circumstances, most people will stick with the default unless it proposes a behaviour change that is totally unpalatable. Sticking with a default might also depend upon whether people perceive that this is the option the persuader is trying to foist on them. This could lead them to reject it. If it is perceived as the option most favoured by most people already, however, those being presented with a default might be inclined to conform to the status quo rather than make a fuss or appear to be non-conformist.

Another element is the number of choice alternatives. Hence, with or without a default format, people might be offered not just two, but three or more options to choose from. In the end, though, a choice is required. An opportunity might be given for an initial choice to be made and trialled before being rejected in favour of a different option. People might also be given advice about the pros and cons of different options or perhaps ratings of these options on different evaluative scales. Choices might also vary in their simplicity or complexity (Thaler et al., 2013). One frequently cited example of a default choice is organ donation. One study found that countries that required citizens to opt out of organ donation rather than opt in to it achieved the greater number of potential donors (Johnson & Goldstein, 2003).

One key finding is that it is important not to give people too many different choices because this can end up demotivating them to make any choice at all. Yet, some choice is needed to persuade people that they are not being forced down a specific choice path against their will. Hence, an optimal number of choices must be construed with that number being determined in part by the complexity of choosing between them. A degree of cognitive effort will be needed weighing up each option and the more complex the attributes on which cognitive judgements are needed, the smaller the optimal number of choice points will be (Johnson et al., 2012).

When people are presented with two options to choose between, presenting one as the default option usually results in it being chosen most often. One well-known example of this effect is choosing whether to become an organ donor. Research showed that signing up for organ donation was twice as great when people had to opt out rather than opt in to it (Johnson & Goldstein, 2003). Even though some people might interpret the use of a default as a blatant attempt to manipulate their behaviour, many will not notice this and will stick with the default option because they cannot be bothered to make the effort to opt out of it (Smith et al., 2013).

Another outcome preference that many people have been shown to display is to opt for short-term benefits and gains over longer-term ones. In this respect, many people have displayed a tendency to be short-sighted in their choice-making (Koehler, 1991; Shu, 2008). This choice bias can be offset by nudging strategies that place more emphasis on viable and attractive longer-term outcomes (Weber et al., 2007). Often, when people are given the opportunity to choose between a relatively small short-term gain and a relatively large long-term gain, they will opt for the former.

One explanation for this phenomenon is that people discount the value of rewards the further into the future they are moved. The rate of reward-value loss can vary from one type of future benefit to another. People can demonstrate a considerable degree of impatience for some outcomes, but less so with others (Ainslie, 1975; Frederick et al., 2002).

Variances can also occur in the way different people perceive over time. For some, an exclusively linear view of time might increase the impatience they feel for rewards that are delayed over extended periods. Others might be capable of breaking down time differently and seeing a one-year delay as manageable psychologically, assuming it is also manageable economically where the reward is in monetary terms and they need the income (Ebert & Prelec, 2007; Scholten & Read, 2010; Zauberman et al., 2009). This effect of short-term versus long-term options can be switched around by offering up the long-term gain first (rather than the more usual short-term gain first) and then requiring individuals to make a fairly speedy decision (Appell et al., 2011).

In relation to the COVID-19 pandemic, governments and policy makers have recognised that public concerns about vaccines are not simply defined by anti-vaxxer activism. There are many people, without an axe to grind on this subject, who exhibited some hesitation about getting vaccinated for understandable reasons. Their uncertainty about vaccines stemmed from safety considerations linked to doubts about whether all the usual quality control procedures had been followed given the pace at which new vaccines had emerged. Some governments considered whether to pass new legislation that would render the spreading of fake news about COVID-19 vaccines an offence. Any such draconian approach to dealing with a serious matter at a time of global crisis needed to be tempered with understanding that even untruthful stories might trigger more reasonable questions about the safety of vaccines. An educational approach to dealing with this was regarded as an optimal solution to responding to any such public doubts (Marco-Franco et al., 2020).

Risk Nudges and Concerns about Safety

Immunisation was highlighted as the eventual escape route from COVID-19 from the point at which epidemiological modellers in Britain first advised the government about the need to deploy comprehensive and wide-ranging NPIs to slow the rate of infections and safeguard hospitals from being overwhelmed by coronavirus patients. This observation might, of course, have contained a lot of truth but it also made a presumption that getting a vaccine out to people would provide the solution needed in the long term. This presumption, however, cannot be taken for granted because it also depends upon public compliance. Producing and distributing a vaccine in sufficient quantities to convenient locations for its administration to the public represented a major logistical challenge, but even if it could be done, it would prove ineffective in large numbers of people simply refused to be vaccinated.

It might seem incredulous to many that anyone would refuse this kind of help, especially if it was presented as the best final solution. Yet, mounting evidence from around the world pointed to growing public scepticism about vaccines, not just for COVID-19, but more generally. This phenomenon was widespread enough that it was becoming increasingly apparent that falling vaccine confidence had already undermined the effectiveness of many immunisation programmes around the world (Cooper et al., 2008; Larson et al., 2014; Omer et al., 2009; Phadke et al., 2016). According to the World Health Organization, the reluctance of take vaccines represented one of the major health threats confronting the world (WHO, 2019).

As news emerged about progress with new vaccines for protect against the new coronavirus, further soundings with the public indicated the presence of some uncertainty about safety. This response was not restricted to anti-vaxxers. There were factions of the wider public that were asking questions about the side effects of new vaccines. These concerns meant that some were inclined to adopt a wait and see policy rather than being first in the queue for protection.

The concerns about the safety of vaccines, however, can be found far beyond anti-vaxxer activism. It also stems not just from a concern about personal safety or the safety of one's children, but can also be attributed to a distrust of authorities, in both health and politics. Hence, even a vaccine that has been passed as safe and ethical might still be rejected by many people on the grounds that they simply do not believe what those in authority say (Roeder, 2020).

Research found that exposure to misinformation about vaccines could reduce people's confidence in new vaccines. Before exposure to the information, over half of those questioned (54%) said they were willing to try a new vaccine. After being shown five false messages about vaccines that had already been circulated widely online, this proportion dropped to 48%.

At the same time, there was a slight increase (from 40% to 42%) in those expressing doubts about a new vaccine. Only a small minority of people said they definitely would not get a vaccine, but even this number increased (6–10%) after exposure to false claims about vaccines (Roeder, 2020).

More generally, large-scale international research conducted under the auspices of the Vaccine Confidence Project monitored public confidence in vaccines in different parts of the world and found that trust in key information sources was important to vaccine acceptance. This study led by Heidi Larson of the London School of Hygiene and Tropical Medicine analysed public confidence in vaccines across 149 countries. Surveys were conducted between 2015 and 2019 that collected data from over 284,000 adults aged 16 and over. Respondents were questioned about a range of matters, but principally, this inquiry was concerned with whether people regarded vaccines as important, safe and effective (de Figueiredo et al., 2020).

Larson and her colleagues combined data from 290 nationally representative surveys to model public perceptions of the safety and effectiveness of vaccines (Larson et al., 2014). Vaccine uptake in each country was also assessed and modelled against demographics, socio-economic factors and degree of trust in different sources of information about immunisation, such as family friends and health professionals. Changes in vaccine safety protocols were also examined for different countries.

Significant declines in public confidence in vaccine safety were found across different parts of the European Union, and especially in Poland (64% agreeing strongly that vaccines were safe in November 2018, dropping to 53% by December 2019). Poland had witnessed an organised anti-vaccine movement at that time. Yet, confidence in the safety of vaccines improved elsewhere, for example, in Finland, France, Italy, Ireland, and the United Kingdom. In the United Kingdom, there was an increase in people saying they strongly agreed that vaccines were safe (from 47% in May 2018 to 52% in November, 2019).

Confidence in vaccines fell between 2015 and 2019 in parts of Asia, especially in Indonesia, the Philippines, Pakistan and South Korea. Confidence in vaccines was found to be especially likely to falter in countries defined by religious extremism and political instability. Although even where confidence seemed to be waning, most people still believed that vaccines were important and effective (Larson et al., 2014). Where public doubts had surfaced, Larsen and her colleagues concluded that this had happened where political leaders had queried the safety of measles, mumps and rubella vaccine. Ultimately, evidence showed that it was the perceived effectiveness of vaccines more than their perceived safety that predicted their uptake. Even in countries not usually rated highly for their political stability, such as Iraq, Liberia and Senegal, over nine in ten people surveyed agreed it was important for children to be vaccinated. A further important finding that also had a bearing on the success of government actions related to COVID-19 was that public trust in health-care workers for medical and health advice was more important than other information sources in increasing the likelihood of vaccine uptake (de Figueiredo et al., 2020).

Hesitancy Nudging through False Narratives

Not everyone was enthusiastic about getting vaccinated. It was true that some countries had been generally more vaccine hesitant than others. Within countries, some population sub-groups displayed hesitancy when others around them did not. The reasons for these differences were often tied to the messages different groups had received from different sources about the efficacy of vaccines and also about their side effects. Some of these beliefs were influenced by clearly false narratives about COVID-19 and its vaccines. Other beliefs were grounded in understandable concerns about vaccines that had been developed much more rapidly than normal. For some people, there remained questions about whether scientists had cut corners to get vaccines developed and approved quickly under pressure from governments.

Yet, in weighing up the evidence about vaccine hesitancy, some people were cautious for perfectly logical reasons based on a lack of relevant scientific evidence to alleviate their concerns. This was true, in particular, of pregnant women, many of whom were cautious about taking COVID vaccines for fear they might harm their unborn child. In the United Kingdom, the Royal College of Obstetricians and Gynaecologists (RCOG) found that 58% of pregnant women offered a vaccine against COVID-19 had refused it. Two-thirds of these women (65%) were worried about the possible side effects of the vaccine on their babies. One problem in countering this viewpoint was that there was not always sufficient science or relevance to reassure pregnant women about COVID vaccines' potential side effects. Pregnant women, as is customary with this kind of development research, had not been included in the original studies that established the efficacy and safety of these vaccines (Perez, 2021).

What did become known was that COVID-19 itself held risks for pregnant women, with one American study showing that they were 14 times as likely as non-pregnant women to die of the disease. COVID-19 had also been found to increase the risk of miscarriage. It was not until February 2021, two months after the first vaccines had been approved, that there were clinical trials with pregnant women. Data eventually accumulated from around the world of pregnant women who got vaccinated even though there had been little research and there have apparently been no increased risks to women or their babies from the vaccine.

Nevertheless, the public health authorities did not really push hard on pregnant women to get vaccinated. Cases of pregnant women being admitted to intensive care with COVID-19 in England, Wales and Northern

Ireland, however, encouraged health authorities to voice a greater sense of urgency for pregnant women to get vaccinated. The lack of clarity over messaging about vaccination of pregnant women understandably left many confused as to the best and safest course of action. This state of affairs also meant that some women were vulnerable to the influences of conspiracy theories about COVID-19 vaccines frequently circulating online.

Conspiracy theories about COVID-19 have been connected to groups that espouse "new age" philosophy. Included among these groups are individuals that are highly visible on the Internet in the health field, especially the well-being and yoga industries. The Centre for Countering Digital Hate (CCDH) conducted research that found that 12 "influencers" produced nearly 70% of online vaccine misinformation. Most of these influencers were associated with the wellness or well-being industries (Kinchen, 2021).

One American wellness "expert", Kelly Brogan posted a video online that rapidly accumulated a large audience in which she claimed that COVID-19 deaths were being increased by fear and that this fear had been stoked to a significant extent by the mainstream media. Lockdown measures were castigated as "dehumanising" and were compared to the Holocaust.

In another investigation into conspiracy groups by a podcaster, Annie Kelly, many of the right-wing promulgators of misleading information about many health issues, including COVID-19, were found to be young women frequently working as online influencers and working in the wellness industries as life coaches or instructors of exercise forms such as *kundalini* yoga. One explanation that has been offered for the role of yoga here is that it does focus very much of the individual and his/her well-being through techniques that involve high degrees of personal control. As such "health" becomes part on one's personal being and needs to be nurtured by the individual through inward looking methods that cultivate a deep knowing of the "self". Collective ideas such as "public" health therefore sit less well with this life philosophy of individualism. The coronavirus and anti-vaxxer conspiracy theories put out by a relatively small number of high-profile online influencers stem therefore from this rejection of an intervention created by and for the "collective".

Social Groups, Public Trust and Vaccination Adoption

Experts in medicine and science repeatedly advised the public that the coronavirus problem was not going to simply go away. It might be many years before the COVID-19 virus could be neutralised through vaccines, prophylactics and effective treatments or more organically via "herd immunity". Given that viruses like this one can evolve over time, treatments for one version of the virus might prove to be ineffective at controlling a new version.

Whether or not people feel they trust official sources from whom advice is received about getting vaccinated might depend in part on whether people identify with those sources. If there is a sense of shared group membership or social identity, this could then encourage message receivers to have more faith in message senders on these matters. Politics has been blamed for undermining public confidence in vaccines for COVID-19.

Research in the United States found a social divide in how people felt about vaccination that was associated with their political allegiances. A survey conducted in September 2021 showed that Americans were polarised in their confidence about a coronavirus vaccine with Democrats being 14 percentage points more likely to take the vaccine than Republicans. There were also significant ethnic differences in willingness to take the vaccine. Black Americans (32%) were far less likely than whites (52%) Hispanics (56%) or Asian Americans (72%) to say they would get vaccinated (Stone, 2020).

Group processes and social identity effects have not always been found to differentiate between public responses to pandemic-related behaviour. One instance of this was found in relation to attitudes towards vaccination. In studies of how people reacted to others who were known to have been vaccinated, no differences of opinion emerged between research participants who had themselves been vaccinated or not vaccinated. In other words, a vaccinated person was liked equally by other vaccinate people and non-vaccinated people (Korn et al., 2020; Weisel, 2021).

Elsewhere, however, social identity was found to affect people's willingness to get vaccinated. The local community received a boost in terms of its relevance to many people during the pandemic. In the face of severe behavioural restrictions, many people turned to their local community for support. In an atmosphere of "we're all in this together" neighbours often spoke to each other for the first time or had an issue to bond over that went beyond the everyday pleasantries that characterised their usual conversations. If local communities could instil in their members a sense of civic responsibility, for example, to get vaccinated, and if individuals in that community identified themselves in terms of being members of this group, community influences could also influence behaviour. One study found that this kind of local community identity increased the tendency of people to show greater willingness to get vaccinated (Wakefield & Khauser, 2021).

Evidence obtained from two small surveys of adults in the United Kingdom indicated that while risks were weighed up by people before deciding to get tested for COVID-19 or get vaccinated against it, social support networks were also important factors that could influence likelihood of taking these self-protective steps (Jaspal & Breakwell, 2021).

Theory of Planned Behaviour and Vaccine Uptake

The theory of planned behaviour was used as a design model for research into people's vaccine hesitancy. There was a great deal of concern about vaccine hesitancy and people could give numerous reasons for not wishing to get inoculated despite the large volumes of public health advice telling them that this was the ultimate safeguard against serious infection. In understanding why people might or might not get vaccinated, it is relevant to find out about the beliefs and attitudes they hold about this behaviour and whether these internal cognitive processes push them towards or away from it.

One American study evaluated public intentions to get a flu vaccine during the 2020–2021 flu season. While public attention was focused on the novel coronavirus, other disease had not gone away, including influenza. Across a sample of 364 adults, one in five (20%), had already had their flu vaccine. Among those who had not done so, there were widespread concerns (among 58%) about adverse effects from the flu vaccine. Those who perceived that the vaccine would be personally beneficial to them were more likely to get vaccinated. As well as these internalised beliefs, subjective norms also had an impact, with those told by their doctors that it would be a good idea for them to get vaccinated, were then more likely to do so (Shmueli, 2021).

Another study in Iran surveyed over 10,000 people and measured a range of psychological constructs, including core constructs of the theory of planned behaviour. Perceived COVID-19 infectability and fear of COVID-19 were also measured. The research found that perceived infectability (i.e., likelihood of being infected with the new virus), perceived behavioural control, subjective norm and attitudes towards vaccination (i.e., positive rather than negative) all predicted intention to get vaccinated. Greater fear of COVID-19 was also related to vaccination intention and added to the impact of the other predictor variables (Yahaghi et al., 2021).

Other research confirmed the results of this study that people's intentions to get a flu vaccine were strengthened when they believed it would be beneficial to them and that it would help to protect others. Many also said they would go to their doctor's office to get vaccinated and this was something within their behavioural control – that is, they were still able to get vaccinated this way, while other would go to their local pharmacy (Jung & Albarracin, 2021; Mercadanate & Law, 2020; Shmueli, 2021).

The theory of planned behaviour can offer theoretical insights into why people might reject a particular course of action. Those not wishing to get vaccinated will generally have internalised concerns about adverse side effects, which can dominate their beliefs about vaccination. Others may also have seen, heard or read other people questioning the safety of vaccines and hence develop perceptions of subjective norms across a wider community that this intervention was being widely avoided (Asciak et al., 2013).

One source of reassurance could be found among those people who had been vaccinated previously without significant ill effects. Not only would they themselves derive confidence that the latest vaccines were, but they might also impact this belief to others and hence enabling it to become a persuasive "subjective norm".

Another barrier to vaccination is a fear of needles. With these people, there may be alternative administration techniques that could be used (Grohskopf et al., 2020). For those saying that getting a vaccine was inconvenient and hence represented a "behaviour control" factor that worked against the uptake of the primary target behaviour, public health officials would need to ensure that there is an ample supply of vaccination centres so that no one would have to travel far to get to one. By getting family members on board with vaccination, more positively disposed subjective norms can be cultivated among an important reference group for those reluctant to get inoculated.

The theory of planned behaviour underpinned the design of research into people's vaccine hesitancy. One American study evaluated public intentions to get a flu vaccine during the 2020–2021 flu season. While public attention was focused on the novel coronavirus, other disease had not gone away, including influenza. Across a sample of 364 adults, one in five (20%) had already had their flu vaccine. Among those who had not done so, there were widespread concerns (among 58%) about adverse effects from the flu vaccine. Those who perceived that the vaccine would be personally beneficial to them were more likely to get vaccinated. As well as these internalised beliefs, subjective norms also had an impact, with those told by their doctors that it would be a good idea for them to get vaccinated, were then more likely to do so (Shmueli, 2021).

Other research confirmed the results of this study that people's intentions to get a flu vaccine were strengthened when they believed it would be beneficial to them and that it would help to protect others. Many also said they would go to their doctor's office to get vaccinated and this was something within their behavioural control – that is, they were still able to get vaccinated this way, while other would go to their local pharmacy (Mercadanate & Law, 2020; Jung & Albarracin, 2021; Schmueli, 2021).

In New Zealand, researchers found that intentions to get vaccinated were strengthened by holding positive attitudes towards it, having trust in the media and by perceptions that others were positively disposed towards it. Knowing more about the vaccine also increased intentions to get inoculated but did not significantly predict eventual vaccination behaviour.

There was plenty of earlier evidence to show that social norms were very important to people getting vaccinated, long before the COVID-19 pandemic (e.g., Juon et al., 2017; Smith-McLallen & Fishbein, 2008; also see Brewer et al., 2017). The significance of this variable as a predictor of vaccination intention was also confirmed during the coronavirus pandemic (Bradshaw et al, 2020; Lee & Su, 2020; Xiao & Borah, 2020). It is especially important that a person's own family or friends are positive about vaccination. These are key reference points for most people (Bish et al., 2011).

The complication during the coronavirus pandemic was that there were so many unknowns about this new disease and that at the outset science was on a steep learning curve (Rimal & Storey, 2020). This meant that people had to trust that scientists knew what they were doing and would find safe solutions to protect them from this new disease. As the primary source of information, it was also important that the mainstream mass media could be trusted to report news about COVID-19 accurately and clearly. While the scientific knowledge may had had gaps in it as the pandemic progressed early on, if sources of that knowledge were trusted, this could put many people's minds at rest. In trying to provide digestible news reports about often very technical scientific and medical topics, it was important that journalists gave information that could be believed and was relevant and usable.

The importance of this trust was underlined by findings that when people had more confidence in the media, they were more likely to get vaccinated (Bradshaw et al., 2020; Cadeddu et al., 2020; de Figueiredo et al., 2020; Liu & Yang, 2020). If trusted media coverage leads to a better-informed public, this, too, can help to encourage populations to get vaccinated (Schulz & Hartung, 2020). Being better informed also meant that any negative attitudes towards vaccination, which might have been cultivated by conspiracy theories, would be countered by internalised scientific understanding (Chen et al., 2020).

Within the theory of planned behaviour, attitudes were hypothesised to drive behavioural intentions. In the context of COVID vaccination, therefore, it was critical that people developed positive attitudes towards vaccines and vaccination. If a person holds the view that getting vaccinated is desirable (i.e., positive attitude), they will be more likely to do so (Binder et al., 2009; Xiao, 2019).

COM-B and Vaccine Adoption

Vaccine hesitancy presented one of the major hurdles to getting populations comprehensively inoculated against COVID-19. Research had already been carried out about vaccination uptake during pandemics before the COVID-19 pandemic. One review of evidence accumulated during the 2009 global influenza pandemic (H1N1) found there was a low uptake of vaccines in many countries. Propensity to get vaccinated was influenced by a number of factors that could act independently or collectively. There were perceptions of the threat posed by the virus. There were also concerns about the safety of the vaccine. In addition, people sometimes made reference to the perspectives of social groups to which they belonged. When people thought that there were others around them that wanted them to get vaccinated, they would be more likely to do so (Bish et al., 2011). This type of influence is recognised by the theory of planned behaviour by its concept of subjective norms. It is also a factor prominently identified by the group processes/social identity perspective.

Vaccine hesitancy, however, was not initially present in regard to the COVID-19 pandemic. In a British study, people were surveyed in October 2019 before the pandemic and again in April 2020 as it had taken hold in their country. By the second wave that occurred during the first national lockdown, more than eight in ten (85%) of respondents and over half (55%) of vaccine sceptics said they would be willing to get vaccinated against COVID-19. Those who perceived greater risk for themselves and their families from COVID-19 were more likely than average to show vaccination willingness. The perception that intensive care units had low availability before the pandemic was associated also with poor trust in medical experts and in due course weaker support for COVID-19 vaccination. Hence, pre-existing attitudes before the pandemic influenced behavioural intentions during it (Blanchard-Rohner et al., 2020).

Another UK study confirmed the positive orientation towards COVID vaccination among most "at-risk" people. When older people (aged 70+) and others across the age spectrum with chronic respiratory disease were questioned about their willingness to receive a COVID-19 vaccine, an overwhelming proportion was affirmative (86%). This intention as backed up in most cases by the perception that COVID-19 could present a health risk for some time and by the view that the risks from COVID-19, that had received much media coverage, were not exaggerated. This study obtained data on a range of other questions and also invited its respondents to write their views about the pandemic in their own words. The Behaviour Change Wheel, one expression of the COM-B model, was used to guide the data analysis (Williams et al., 2020).

The timing of this research in April 2020 was significant because this was during the very early stage of the UK lockdown. This showed that the willingness to get vaccinated as the pandemic first became established was already strong among people at greatest risk from this new disease and that such individuals were likely to respond positively to campaigns presenting them with messages that made them feel empowered and therefore capable and created environmental conditions that would facilitate (i.e., provide the opportunity for) adoption of a specific protective behaviour (in this case, getting vaccinated). At the same time, it was also apparent from the findings that there was still a sizeable proportion of people, among those designated as greatest risk of serious illness and death from COVID-19 who harboured doubts about getting vaccinated or were, as yet, undecided about what to do.

There was further evidence of spin-off benefits of COVID-19 on public orientations towards getting vaccinated in general with nearly four in ten of the respondents to this survey (38%) saying that it would now make them more likely to get an annual flu jab and even more (51%) saying the same about getting vaccinated against pneumonia (Williams et al., 2020).

In an alternative approach to investigating explanations of vaccination intent, Twitter posts were used instead of self-reports to measure people's orientations towards COVID-19 vaccines. Tweets were analysed for their references to capability, opportunity and motivation factors, as outlined in the COM-B (capability, opportunity, motivation behaviour) model. In an analysis of 5,000 tweets about COVID-19 across November 2020, it was found that those conveying a negative intention to get vaccinated ($n = 182$) outnumbered those with a positive intent ($n = 97$). Using relational statistics, tweets linked to capability, opportunity and motivation were more likely to be associated also with tweets expressing negative intentions to get vaccinated (Liu & Liu, 2021).

Lessons about Vaccination

Vaccination against COVID-19 was regarded as the critical intervention from the start of the pandemic. Huge investment in vaccine development significantly shortened the usual timeframe over which this would normally take place. That achievement in itself proved also to be a factor in discouraging some people from getting vaccinated. Vaccination rates varied significantly between countries at different time points in the global vaccination effort. Some countries had proved more effective than others in their vaccine procurement strategies. Some countries were at the forefront of vaccine development and therefore had their own supplies to draw upon. In addition, national populations varied in their anti-vaxxer sentiments. There were many conspiracy stories about vaccines in circulation that discouraged some people from getting inoculated because they were suspicious that the vaccines presented health risks because of their ingredients, or in the belief that they had not been thoroughly safety checked, or quite simply because they were seen as instruments of some hidden agenda of public control. As evidence reviewed at the top of this chapter indicated, anti-vaxxer sentiments were already well-established in some communities.

As successive waves of COVID-19 rose and fell in different countries, some governments had been encouraged by successful vaccination programmes to ride them out, as their death rates and hospitalisation levels remained low, while others for which this was not the case, re-introduced unpopular behavioural restrictions, sometimes triggering civil disturbances. Some governments threatened to make vaccination against COVID-19 mandatory. Other countries felt that such draconian measures would be difficult to implement in practice and would cause ever more powerful public resentment and psychological reactance against it.

This chapter has indicated that a number of psychological models were utilised during the pandemic to underpin research into public participation in vaccination programmes and each of these models – nudge theory, social identity theory, theory of planned behaviour and the COM-B model – yielded research evidence to show how public willingness to get vaccinated can be achieved through subtle behavioural triggering and persuasion techniques. At the time of writing, it remains to be seen whether governments will follow through with threats to force vaccination on their populations. The review of psychology-based research into the design and impact measurement of more or less draconian methods of behaviour change has shown that both types of interventions can be useful to achieve public compliance with protective and preventive interventions to combat COVID-19.

The challenge is to find which interventions and combination of interventions are likely to work best under the prevailing circumstances.

References

Ahmed, W., Vidal-Alaball, J., Downing, J., & Segul, F. L. (2020). COVID-19 and the 5G conspiracy theory: Social network analysis of Twitter data. *Journal of Medical Internet Research, 22*(5), e19458.

Ainslie, G. (1975). Specious reward: A behavioral theory of impulsiveness and impulse control. *Psychological Bulletin, 82*(4), 463–496.

Allington, D., Duffy, B., Wessely, S., Dhavan, N., & Rubin, J. (2020). Health-protective behaviour, social media usage and conspiracy belief during the COVID-19 public health emergency. *Psychological Medicine, 51*(10), 1–7.

Appell, K. C., Hardity, D. J., & Weber, E. U. (2011). Asymmetric discounting of gains and losses: A query theory account. *Journal of Risk and Uncertainty, 43*(2), 107–126.

Asciak, R., Balzan, M., & Buttgieg, J. (2013). Predictors of seasonal influenza vaccination in chronic asthma. *Multidisciplinary Respiratory Medicine, 8*(68), 1–6, https://doi.org/10.1186/2049-6958-8-68

Binder, A. R., Dalrymple, K. E., Brossard, D., & Scheufele, D. A. (2009). The soul of a polarized democracy: Testing theoretical linkages between talk and attitude extremity during the 2004 presidential election. *Communication Research, 36*(3), 315–340. https://doi.org/10.1177/0093650209333023

Bish, A., Yardley, L., Nicoll, A., & Michie, S. (2011). Factors associated with uptake of vaccination against pandemic influenza: A systematic review. *Vaccine, 29*(38), 6472– 6484. https://doi.org/10.1016/j.vaccine.2011.06.107

Blakely, R. (2020, 13th November). Herd immunity put at risk by a few lies about vaccine *The Times*, 11.

Blanchard-Rohner, G., Caprettini, B., Rohner, D., & Voth, H. (2020). Impact of COVID-19 and health system performance on vaccination hesitancy: Evidence from a two-leg representative survey in the UK. *SSRN.* https://doi.org/10.2139/ssrn.3627335

Bradshaw, A. S., Shelton, S. S., Wollney, E., Treise, D., & Auguste, K. (2020). Pro-vaxxers get out: Anti-vaccination advocates influence undecided first-time, pregnant, and new mothers on Facebook. *Health Communication.* 1–10. https://doi.org/10.1080/10410236.2020.1712037

Brewer, N. T., Chapman, G. B., Rothman, A. J., Leask, J., & Kempe, A. (2017). Increasing vaccination: Putting psychological science into action. *Psychological Science Public Interest*, *18*(3), 149–207. doi: 10.1177/1529100618760521

Cadeddu, C., Daugbjerg, S., Ricciardi, W., & Rosano, A. (2020). Beliefs towards vaccination and trust in the scientific community in Italy. *Vaccine*, *38*(42), 6609–6617. https://doi.org/10.1016/j.vaccine.2020.07.076

Chen, L., Zhang, Y., Young, R., Wu, X., & Zhu, G. (2020). Effects of vaccine-related conspiracy theories on Chinese young adults' perceptions of the HPV vaccine: An experimental study. *Health Communication*. 1–11. https://doi.org/1 0.1080/10410236.2020.1751384

Cooper, L. Z., Larson, H. J., & Katz, L. (2008). Protecting public trust in immunization. *Pediatrics*, *122*, 149–153.

de Figueiredo, A., Simas, C., Karafillakis, E., Peterson, P., & Larson, H. J. (2020). Mapping global trends in vaccine confidence and investigating barriers to vaccine uptake: A large-scale retrospective temporal modelling study. *The Lancet*, *396*(10255), 898–908.

Ebert, J. E., & Prelec, D. (2007). The fragility of time: Time-insensitivity and valuation of the near and far future. *Management Science*, *53*(9), 1423–1438.

Edridge, A. W. D., Kaczorowska, J., Hoste, A. C. R., Bakker, M., Klein, M., Loens, K., Jebbink, M. F. et al. (2020). *Nature Medicine*, *26*(11), 1691–1693. https://doi.org/ 10.1038/s41591-020-1083-1

Frederick, S., Loewenstein, G., & O'Donoghue, T. (2002). Time discounting and time preference: A critical review. *Journal of Economic Literature*, *40*(2), 351–401.

Goodwin, M. (2016). In A. Kemmerer, C. Mollers, M. Steinbeis, & G. Wagner. (Eds.), *Choice Architecture in Democracies: Exploring the Legitimacy of Nudging. Architecture, Choice Architecture and Dignity*. (pp. 285–307). Baden-Baden/Oxford: Nomos/Hart Publishing.

Grohskopf, L. A. Liburd, L. C., & Redfield, R. R. (2020). Addressing influenza vaccination disparities during the COVID-19 pandemic. *JAMA*, *324*(11), 1029–1030. https://doi.org/10.1001/jama.2020.15845

Harrison, E. A., & Wu, J. W. (2020). Vaccine confidence in the time of COVID-19. *European Journal of Epidemiology*, 22th April, 1–5. Available at: https://www.ncbi.nlm.nih.gov/pmc/articles/PMC7174145/

Iwasaki, A. (2020). What reinfections mean for COVID-19. *The Lancet Infectious Disease*, *21*:3–5. Retrieved from: https://www.thelancet.com/pdfs/journals/laninf/PIIS1473-3099(20)30783-0.pdf

Jaspal, R., & Breakwell, G. M. (2021). Social support, perceived risk and the likelihood of COVID-19 testing and vaccination: Cross-sectional data from the United Kingdom. *Current Psychology*, *8*, 1–13. https://doi.org/10.1007/s12144-021-01681-z

Johnson, E. J., & Goldstein, D.G. (2003). Do defaults save lives? *Science*, *302*(5649), 1338–1339.

Johnson, E. J., Shu, S. B., Dellaert, B. G. C., Fox, C., Goldstein, D. G., Haeubl, G., Larrick, R. P., Payne, J. W., Schkade, D., Wansink, B., & Weber, E. U. (2012). Beyond nudges: Tools of a choice architecture. *Marketing Letters*, *23*(2), 487–504.

Juon, H.-S., Rimal, R. N., Klassen, A., & Lee, S. (2017). Social norm, family communication, and HBV screening among Asian Americans. *Journal of Health Communication*, *22*(12), 981–989. https://doi.org/10.1080/10810730.2017.1388454

Jung, H., & Albarracin, D. (2021). Concerns for others increase the likelihood of vaccination against influenza and COVID-19 more in sparsely rather than densely populated areas. *Proceedings of the National Academy of Science*, USA, *118*(1), e2007538118. https://doi.org/10.1073/pnas.2007538118

Kinchen, R. (2021, 29th August). Downward dog to antivax: Trendy yoga is starting to stretch the truth. *The Sunday Times*, 30.

Koehler, D. J. (1991). Explanation, imagination and confidence in judgement. *Psychological Bulletin, 110*(3), 499–519.

Korn, L., Böhm, R., Meier, N. W., & Betsch, C. (2020). Vaccination as a social contract. *Proceedings of the National Academy of Science USA, 117*(26), 14890–14899.

Larson, H. J., Jarrett, C., Eckersberger, E., Smith, D. M. D., & Paterson, P. (2014). Understanding vaccine hesitancy around vaccines and vaccination from a global perspective: A systematic review of published literature, 2007-2012. *Vaccine, 32*, 2150–2159.

Liu, S., & Liu, J. (2021). Understanding behavioral intentions toward COVID-19 vaccines: Theory-based content analysis of tweets. *Journal of Medical Internet Research, 23*(5), e28118. https://doi.org/10.2196/28118

Liu, Z., & Yang, J. Z. (2020). In the wake of scandals: How media use and social trust influence risk perception and vaccination intention among Chinese parents. *Health Communication*, 1–12. https://doi.org/10.1080/10410236.2020.1748834

Mahase, E. (2020). Vaccinating the UK: How the Covid vaccine was approved and other questions answered. *BMJ, 371*, m4759. https://doi.org/10.1136/bmj.m4759

Marco-Franco, J. E., Pita-Barros, P., Vivas-Orts, D., Gonzalez-de-Julian, S., & Vivas-Consuela, D. (2020). COVID-19, fake news and vaccines: Should regulation be implemented? *International Journal of Environmental Research and Public Health, 18*(2), 744. https://doi.org/10.3390/ijerph18020744

Mercadanate, A. R., & Law, V. (2020). Will they, or won't they? Examining patients' vaccine intention for flu and COVID-19 using the Health Belief Model. *Research in Social and Administrative Pharmacy, 17*(9), 1596–1605. https://doi.org/10.1016/j.sapharm.2020.12.012

Omer, S. D., Salmon, D. A., Orenstein, W. A., & Halsey, N. (2009). Vaccine refusal, mandatory immunization, and the risks of vaccine-preventable diseases. *New England Journal of Medicine, 360*, 1981–1988.

Perez, C. C. (2021, 29th August). Pregnant women are Covid's invisible victims. *The Sunday Times*, 26.

Phadke, V. K., Bednarczyk, R. A., Salmon, D. A., & Omer, S. B. (2016). Association between vaccine refusal and vaccine-preventable diseases in the United States: A review of measles and pertussis. *Journal of the American Medical Association, 315*, 1149–1158.

Rimal, R. N., & Storey, J. D. (2020). Construction of meaning during a pandemic: The forgotten role of social norms. *Health Communication, 35*(14), 1732–1734. doi: 10.1080/10410236.2020.1838091

Roeder, A. (2020, 20th July). Social solidarity and widespread public trust needed to boost vaccine confidence during COVID-19. Harvard University. Available at: https://www.hsph.harvard.edu/news/features/vaccine-confidence-social-solidarity-covid19/

Scheibehenne, B., Greifeneder, R., & Todd, P. (2010). Can there ever be too many options: A meta-analytic review of choice overload. *Journal of Consumer Research*, 37(3), 409–425.

Scholten, M., & Read, D. (2010). The psychology of intertemporal tradeoffs. *Psychological Review*, 117(3), 925–944.

Shmueli, L. (2021). Predicting intention to receive COVID-19 vaccine among the general population using the health belief model and the theory of planned behavior model. *BMC Public Health*, 21, 804. https://doi.org/10.1186/s12889-021-10816-7

Shu, S. B. (2008). Future-biased search: The quest for the ideal. *Journal of Behavioral Decision Making*, 21(4), 52–377.

Schulz, P. J., & Hartung, U. (2020). Unsusceptible to social communication? The fixture of the factors predicting decisions on different vaccinations. *Health Communication*, 36(12). https://doi.org/10.1080/10410236.2020

Smith, M. (2021, 15th January). International study: How many people will take the COVID vaccine? YouGov. Retrieved from: https://yougov.co.uk/topics/health/articles-reports/2021/01/15/international-study-how-many-people-will-take-covi

Smith, N. C., Goldstein, D., & Johnson, E. (2013). Choice without awareness: Ethical and policy implications of defaults. *Journal of Public Policy*, 32(2), 159–172.

Smith-McLallen, A., & Fishbein, M. (2008). Predictors of intentions to perform six cancer-related behaviours: Roles for injunctive and descriptive norms. *Psychology, Health & Medicine*, 13(4), 389–401. https://doi.org/10.1080/13548500701842933

Stone, J. (2020, 23rd September). Public trust in COVID-19 vaccines is being eroded by politics. *Forbes*. Available at: https://www.forbes.com/sites/judystone/2020/09/23/public-trust-in-covid-19-vaccines-are-being-eroded-by-politics/?sh=20aa7b2c1534

Thaler, R. H., Sunstein, C. R., & Balz, J. P. (2013). Choice architecture. In E. Shafir (Ed.), *The Behavioral Foundations of Public Policy* (pp. 428–439). Princeton, NJ: Princeton University Press.

The Lancet. (2021). COVID-19 vaccines: The pandemic will not end overnight. 2(1), E1. Retrieved from: https://www.thelancet.com/journals/lanmic/article/PIIS2666-5247(20)30226-3/fulltext

Wakefield, J. R. H., & Khauser, A. (2021). Doing it for us: Community identification predicts willingness to receive a COVID-19 vaccination via perceived sense of duty to the community. *Journal of Community and Applied Social Psychology*. https://doi.org/10.1002/casp.2542

Weber, E. U., Johnson, E. J., Milch, K. F., Chang, H., Brodscholl, J. C., & Goldstein, D. G. (2007). Asymmetric discounting in intertemporal choice: A Query-Theory account. *Psychological Science*, 18(6), 516–523.

Weisel, O. (2021). Vaccination as a social contract: The case of COVID-19 and US political partisanship. *Proceedings of the National Academy of Science USA*, 118(13), e2026745118. doi: 10.1073/pnas.2026745118

WHO. (2019). Top then threats to global health in 2019. Available at: https://www.who.int/news-room/feature-stories/ten-threats-to-global-health-in-2019

Williams, L., Gallant, A. J., Rasmussen, S., Brown Nicholls, L. A., Cogan, N., Deakin, K., Young, D., & Flowers, P. (2020). Towards intervention development to increase the uptake of COVID-19 vaccination among those at high risk: Outlining evidence-based and theoretically informed future intervention content. *British Journal of Health Psychology*, 25(4), 1039–1054.

Xiao, X. (2019). Follow the heart or the mind? Examining cognitive and affective attitude on HPV vaccination intention. *Atlantic Journal of Communication*, 1–13. https://doi.org/10.1080/15456870.2019.1708743

Xiao, X., & Borah, P. (2020). Do norms matter? Examining norm-based messages in HPV vaccination promotion. *Health Communication*, 1–9. https://doi.org/10.1080/10410236.2020.1770506

Yahaghi, R., Ahmadizade, S., Fotuhi, R., Taherkhani, E., Ranjbaran, M., Buchali, Z., Jafari, R., Zamani, N., Shahbazkhania, A., Simiari, H., Rahmani, J., Yazdi, N., Alijani, H., Poorzolfaghar, L., Rajabi, F., Lin, C. Y., Broström, A., Griffiths, M. D., & Pakpour, A. H. (2021). Fear of COVID-19 and perceived COVID-19 infectability supplement Theory of Planned Behavior to explain Iranians' intention to get COVID-19 vaccinated. *Vaccines (Basel)*, 9(7), 684. https://doi.org/10.3390/vaccines9070684

YouGov. (2021, 6th January). Boris Johnson has said the rate of Covid-19 vaccination will be increased to 2 million a week in coming weeks. *How likely or unlikely do you think it is that this increase will be achieved?* Retrieved from: https://yougov.co.uk/topics/politics/survey-results/daily/2021/01/06/7ad66/1

YouGov. (2021, 12th January). *COVID-19: Willingness to be vaccinated*. Retrieved from: https://yougov.co.uk/topics/international/articles-reports/2021/01/12/covid-19-willingness-be-vaccinated

Zauberman, G., Kim, B. K., Malkoc, S. A., & Bettman, J. R. (2009). Discounting time and time discounting: Subjective time perception and intertemporal preferences. *Journal of Marketing Research*, 46(4), 543–556.

Index

Printed in the United States
by Baker & Taylor Publisher Services

Printed in the United States
by Baker & Taylor Publisher Services